Discover Superfoods #2

21 Best Superfood Smoothie Recipes

"Super nutrition in 21 delicious smoothie recipes designed to boost energy, improve gut health, and increase mental clarity."

Donna Davidson
&
Kay Wood

DISCLAIMER

Any references to the health benefits of superfood ingredients in this recipe book are the opinions of the authors, based on the best data currently available to them, and are provided for informational purposes only; they are not intended as medical advice.

If you have an existing medical condition and/or concerns about eating any of the ingredients mentioned in this book, you should seek the advice of a qualified medical practitioner before doing so.

* * *

However, recipes are for sharing and the authors are quite happy for you to share individual recipes with your friends – especially if you recommend this book series.

ISBN: 978-0-473-36730-5

THANK YOU GIFT
FROM DONNA & KAY

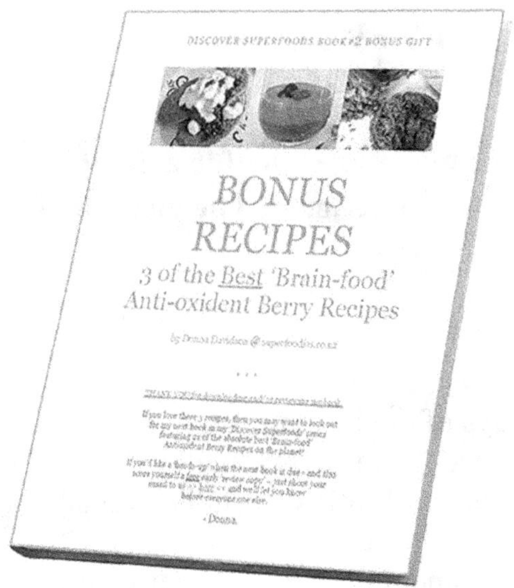

As a reward for getting our book, we'd like to give you

<u>3 FREE BERRY BRAIN-FOOD RECIPES</u>

[Yes, they're Superfood Recipes!]

They're a taste of our 3rd book,
'21 Best Brain-food Berry Recipes'
- Discover Superfoods #3 – <u>available on Amazon.</u>

<< GET YOUR FREE RECIPES HERE >>

Type this into your Internet browser:
www. superfoodies.co.nz/book2free

We think you'll <u>like</u> them!

What did *you* have for breakfast?

Can a morning smoothie actually help you feel better and be healthier?

Good question.

Gone are the days of the ‘nutritionally void’ cup of tea and piece of toast for breakfast! Instead, say ‘hello’ to 21 delicious, nutrient-rich smoothies that will satiate even the best appetites.

These superfood smoothies are especially designed to nourish our organs, cells and immune systems to help keep us safe from health irritations and diseases. They will charge your energy and help slow your body’s degeneration from the aging process.

For ‘superfood newbies’, I usually recommend starting with a daily green smoothie (or at least 5 days a week) to ensure you adequately alkalise your digestive system, in order to receive the best nutrition to charge your body for a healthy, happy and energy-enhanced day.

Whether you found this book through my first book, '21 Best Cacao Recipes', or you're a member of my on-line community on Facebook, or you're hooking up with me here for the first time; I'd like to welcome you to this introduction to the wonderful world of 'superfood smoothies'. It's a very special world to me, because it's the place where my own true health journey began.*

**If you’d like to, you can read my personal story about how finding out that I had dangerously high cholesterol levels led me to* *discover the power of Nature's superfoods, and how they changed my life. See* >> *Pg.54, 'Donna's High Cholesterol Story'.*]

In this book ...

You'll experience the pleasures of 21 completely different and delicious superfood smoothies, as well as my quick-and-easy recipes - simplified over time to be fast and simple to make, while retaining a careful balance of super-nutritious ingredients that will deliver *all* the health-promoting benefits you're looking for.

I invite you to share my daily journey to better health ...

All you have to do is, add these 21 delicious superfood smoothies into your regular diet. Daily, if you want the best results.

If you're like me, looking to boost your brain, body and immune system with some powerful support as they age, I'm sure you'll be pleasantly surprised by the benefits you'll experience in them over the next few months.

In fact, these smoothies may *change* your life!

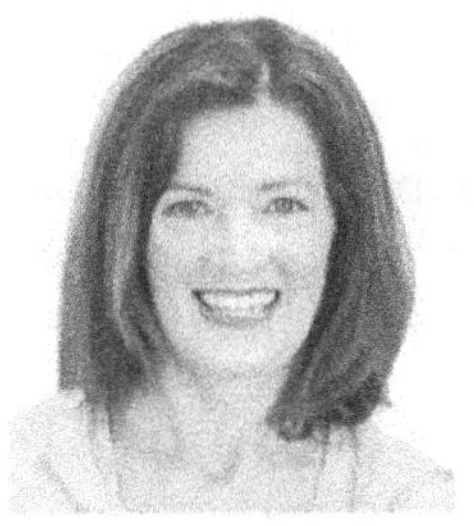

Your Very Good Health,

Donna

Donna Davidson
November, 2016.

* * *

FOLLOW :: Donna on Facebook :: Facebook.com/SuperFoodies

Meet the Authors …

Donna Davidson

Living happily by the Pacific Ocean in beautiful New Zealand, Donna's primary passion has always been in the health, fitness and well-being arena. Several years ago, while working in the superfoods industry, Donna personally experienced the profound benefits of incorporating superfoods into her regular diet and she now credits them with … Read more on pg.52

Kay Wood

Originally from the world of advertising and marketing, Kay has more recently specialised in copywriting and content creation for the Internet. For nearly 10 years Kay has been 'ghost-writing' info blogs for online businesses and offering help to clients struggling to turn their awkward prose and bad spelling into simple and easily understood … Read more on pg.56

Meet the Real Smoothies …

Top 10 Health Benefits of Superfood Smoothies

There are probably more, but these are my top 10:
1. The blending process of smoothies helps to pre-digest food, which makes it easier for the digestive system to break down foods. This is extremely beneficial for those with already compromised digestive systems … Read more on pg.48

What are Superfoods?

Superfoods are a special category of foods found in nature. These foods are superior sources of the anti-oxidants and essential nutrients that our bodies need, but cannot make themselves. Superfoods are calorie-sparse and nutrient-dense, so they pack a lot of punch for their weight and deliver … Read more on pg.58

Superfoods Descriptions + Info

Sacha Inchi Protein Powder: Vegetable protein powder from the South American Sacha Inchi seed. Contains 60% complete protein, all essential amino acids as well as the omega essential fatty acids. Easily digestible and light nutty flavour. Perfect for pre and post workout smoothies, maintaining … Read more on pg.60

Testimonials about Superfoods

Lost over 7kg and feeling so much better: Thank you so much for the healthy delicious treats for Christmas. *(See pg.8 of our first book, '21 Best Superfood Cacao Recipes'.)* I am still enjoying my new eating regime with super foods. I have lost over 7kg and feeling so much better in myself … Read more on pg.64

Meet the Real Proof …

Will, so-called, 'superfoods' really help me become healthier and feel better? Consider the vital relationship between our modern diet and our health: the steady and observable decline in health and rise of chronic conditions such as allergies, asthma, and skin conditions in western countries over the last 60-100 years is generally agreed, by scientists and … Read more on pg.78

Try the Chocolate Pudding Challenge …

The proof is in the pudding.

In our experience, most people find after adding superfoods to their regular diet (often by simply replacing breakfast with a 'superfood smoothie') that they feel more energetic, start noticing improvements or even the elimination of … Read full 'Chocolate Pudding Challenge' on pg.81

* * *

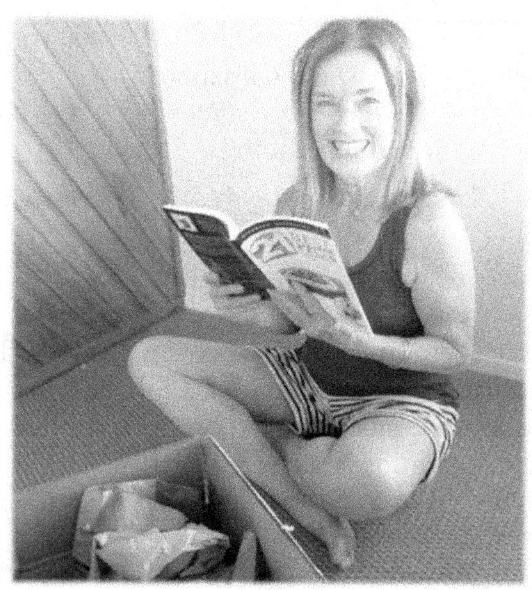

Dreaming of writing your own book?

Many people spend years wanting to write
a book but never do … Why?

How did *we* manage it?

We found a great online writers group, called 'Self-Publishing School'. They provided coaching, training, support, and a step-by-step plan to publishing our first book in 90 days, guaranteed.

They also showed us how to format, upload, and successfully market our book. They involved us in a supportive Facebook community of fellow writers who gave immediate feedback and positive advice all along the way. We had a great experience, and our books have all made it to No.1 on Amazon, so we happily commend SPS to you.

If you believe you have a book in you, but need a little help giving birth to it, check out the Self-Publishing School at the link below:

Self-Publishing School -
http://superfoodies.co.nz/sps

PHOTO Opposite left: The joy of a new author seeing her book in print for the first time!

ACKNOWLEDGMENTS

Special Thanks to ::

The Self-Publishing School gang, especially Chandler Bolt and Sean Sumner. Without your amazing coaching and easy step-by-step plan, this book would probably never exist. We are indebted to you.

We totally recommend Self-Publishing School ::
http://superfoodies.co.nz/sps

Photo Contributors :: Jess Thomson, Donna Davidson
Graphic Design, Layout, Copywriting :: Kay Wood
Recipe Creation + Testing :: Donna Davidson
Mobi / Kindle Formatting :: Jay Syder

Published by ::
Super Healthy Kiwi Publishing

Contact the authors by Snail Mail ::
SuperFoodies NZ
267a Harbour Road
Ohope Beach 3121
New Zealand

Email :: info@superfoodies.co.nz
Website :: http://superfoodies.co.nz
Facebook :: facebook.com/superfoodies.co.nz

Table of Contents

A. BERRY SMOOTHIE RECIPES

B. GREEN SMOOTHIE RECIPES

C. DECADENT SMOOTHIE RECIPES

WHERE TO START?

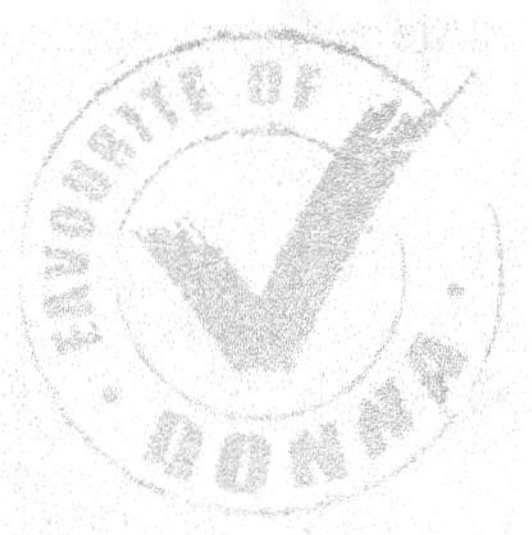

TRY ME!

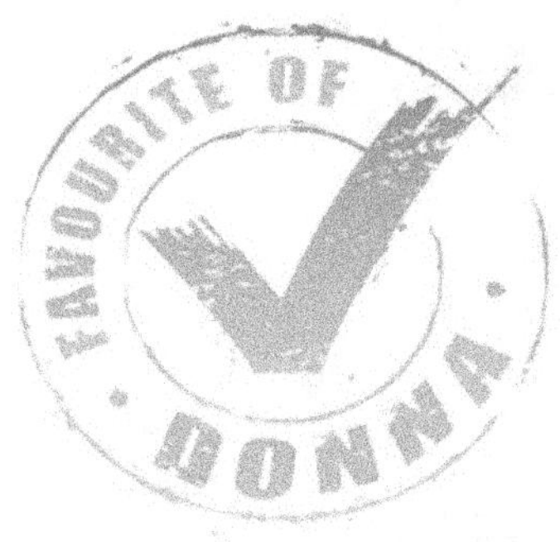

Not sure which recipe to try first?

They all look good, right?

We've made it easy for you. We'll give you a 'tick start'.
The above '**tick**' icon appears next to 3 recipes
personally recommended by Donna.

Donna's Top 3
'Tick Start' Recipes!

1. **Hi-Antioxidant Berry Smoothie** >> TRY ME on pg.8
2. **Big Vit C Smoothie** >> TRY ME on pg.28
3. **Mango Smoothie** >> TRY ME on pg.26

You can't go wrong. It's as easy as 1,2,3 …

"So, do yourself a huge favour, rush and grab your ingredients and easily whip up the healthiest, most delicious smoothie you've ever tasted."

– Donna.

[If you need to order ingredients, it'll take longer, but please don't let that side-track you from beginning this simple first step on your superfood smoothie journey to better health.]

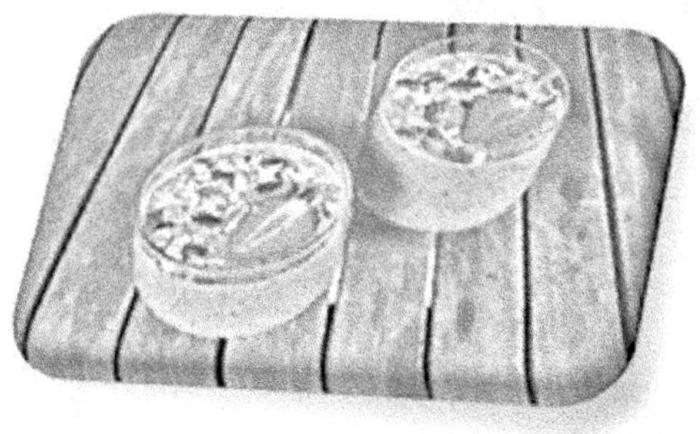

SECTION A

BERRY SMOOTHIE recipes

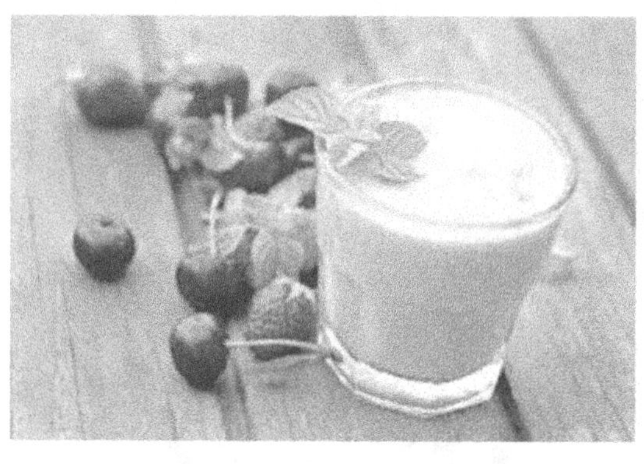

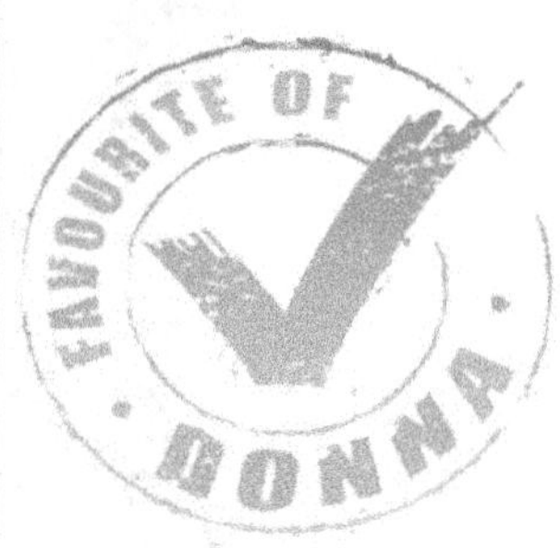

A1. Berry Cocktail Smoothie

Serving size: makes 2 smoothies
Time to make: 10 minutes

Ingredients

1-2 cups fresh mixed berries / or frozen berries
2 frozen bananas, skin removed and chopped
1 handful of fresh mint leaves
2 limes - juice and flesh
2 cups of filtered water / or coconut water
2 teaspoons maqui berry powder / or acai berry powder
1 tablespoon sacha inchi protein powder
1 tablespoon lucuma powder / or yacon powder

Method

1. Place banana, mint leaves, lime juice and flesh, in the blender with some of the water and blitz until well processed.
2. Add the berries, maqui berry powder, sacha inchi and lucuma with the remaining water.
3. Blitz to a smooth texture.

4. Pour into glasses and enjoy.

* Notes:

The limes and mint add a very fresh twist to this delicious berry smoothie.

NEXT Berry Smoothie recipe:
| A2 | Berry Goji Smoothie | Pg.4

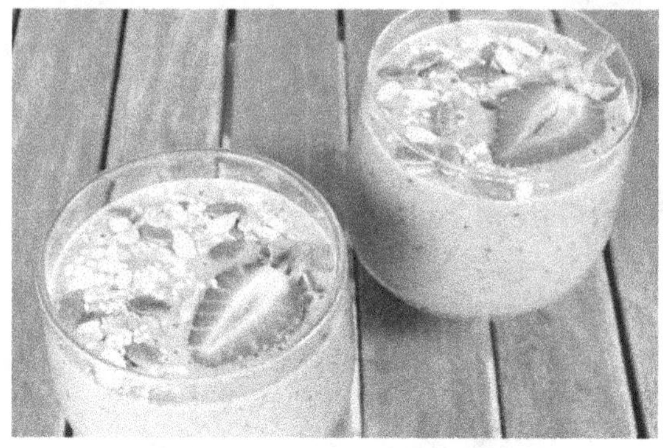

A2. Berry Goji Smoothie

Serving size: makes 2 smoothies
Time to make: 10 minutes

Ingredients

2 cups fresh / or frozen mixed berries
2 large oranges
2 tablespoons goji berries
2 cups of filtered water / or coconut water
2 teaspoons maqui berry powder / or acai berry powder
1 tablespoon sacha inchi protein powder
1 tablespoon lucuma powder
1 tablespoon chia seeds
½ teaspoon of vanilla paste / or extract

Method

1. Peel and chop oranges leaving some white pith on.
2. Place all ingredients into a blender.
3. Blitz until all the fresh fruit is processed to a smooth texture.

4. Pour into glasses and enjoy.

* Notes:

Goji berries have all the essential amino acids and have a reputation as an anti-aging food. I love the taste of them especially together with orange.

Allow a few minutes for the dried berries to rehydrate, the flavour is more intense that way.

NEXT Berry Smoothie recipe:
| A3 | Blueberry Smoothie | Pg.6

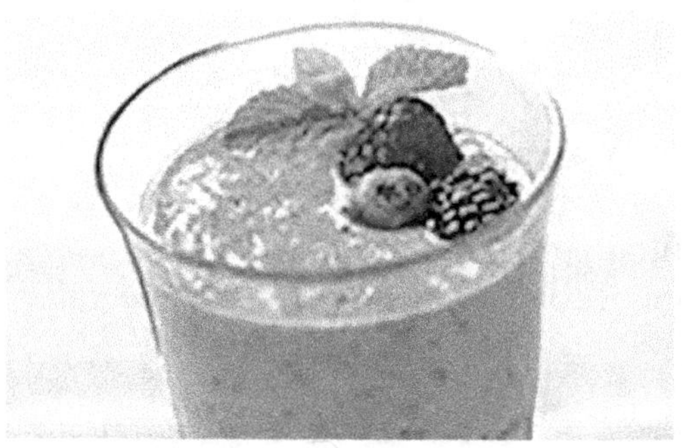

A3. Blueberry Smoothie

Serving size: makes 2 smoothies
Time to make: 10 minutes

Ingredients

1-2 cups fresh / or frozen blueberries
2 frozen bananas, skin removed, chopped
2 cups almond milk / or milk of your choice / or coconut water
2 teaspoons maqui berry powder / or acai berry powder
1 tablespoon sacha inchi protein powder
1 tablespoon lucuma powder
1 tablespoon chia seeds

Method

1. Place all ingredients into a blender.
2. Blitz until all the fresh fruit is processed to a smooth texture.
3. Pour into glasses and enjoy.

* Notes:

According to Dr Oz (from TV's Dr Oz show), lucuma is an 'energy stabilizer' and since lucuma has a low glycaemic index, this is logical. Blueberries naturally are higher in fruit sugars than other berries so lucuma is a great companion in this smoothie.

NEXT Berry Smoothie recipe:
| A4 | High Antioxidant Berry Smoothie | Pg.8

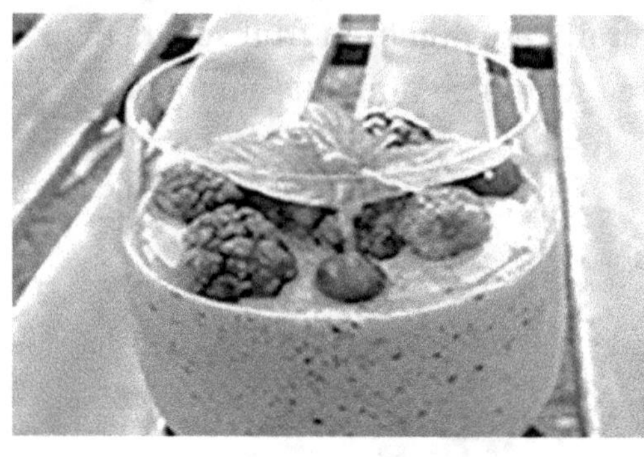

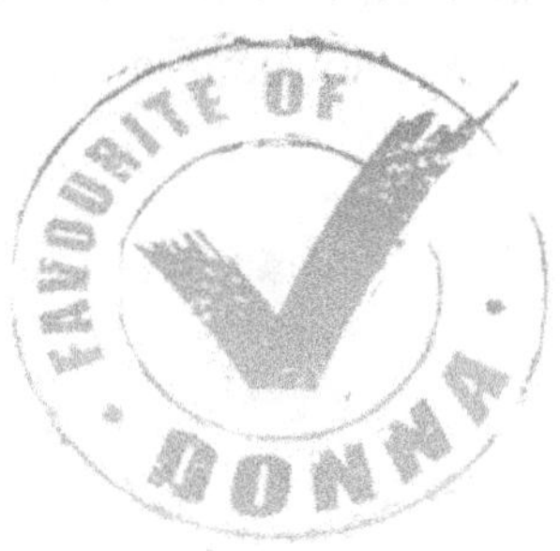

A4. High Antioxidant Berry Smoothie

Serving size: makes 2 smoothies
Time to make: 10 minutes

Ingredients

1 cup mixed fresh / frozen berries (blueberry, blackberry, raspberry or your own combination)
1 frozen banana (skin removed) – chopped
½ cup fresh pineapple
2 cups almond milk / milk of your choice / coconut water
2 teaspoons maqui berry powder / or acai berry powder
2 tablespoons sacha inchi protein powder
1 tablespoon chia seeds

Method

1. Place all ingredients into a blender.
2. Blitz until all fresh fruit is processed to a smooth texture.
3. Pour into glasses and enjoy.

* Notes:

If you don't happen to have fresh berries available, you can double the maqui berry or acai berry powders. It makes this Berry Smoothie very convenient to prepare when travelling.

You can also add 2 teaspoons of our fermented greens powder to aid digestion and boost the nutrient uptake.

NEXT Berry Smoothie recipe:
| A5 | Pomegranate Berry Delight Smoothie | Pg.10

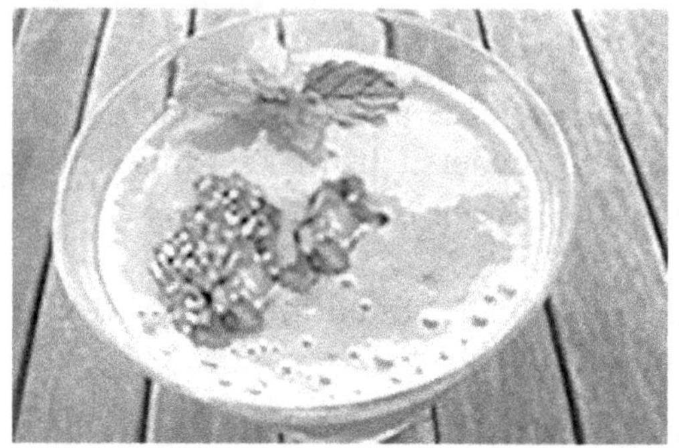

A5. Pomegranate Berry Delight Smoothie

Serving size: makes 2 smoothies
Time to make: 10 minutes

Ingredients

1 cup fresh / or frozen raspberries
1 cup fresh / or frozen blueberries
1 cup pomegranate seeds
1 frozen banana
6 medjool dates / or 8 dried chopped dates
2 cups filtered water / or coconut water
1 tablespoon sacha inchi protein powder
1 tablespoon maca powder
2 teaspoons acai berry powder

Method

1. If using dried dates, let them soak a few minutes in some of the water.
2. Place dates, frozen banana and water into a blender.
3. Blitz until well processed.

4. Add raspberries, blueberries, pomegranate seeds, sacha inchi, maca and acai berry powder to blender; then blitz until well processed and smooth.
5. Pour into glasses and enjoy.

* Notes:

Pomegranates are new for me but I am totally fascinated with them, now that I've learned how to easily remove the seeds. (I treat it like a lemon, cut in half and squeeze or use a lemon squeezer.)

There is not a lot of reliable nutritional information on pomegranates, but their colour alone tells us it is high in antioxidants. This means they are good for heart health and cellular protection.

Protein powder is an important element in smoothies: it helps carry the sugars to even out the glycaemic load. Protein supports our immune system, our metabolism and helps our bodies to sustain lean muscle.

NEXT Berry Smoothie recipe:

| A6 | Strawberry Date Surprise Smoothie | Pg.12

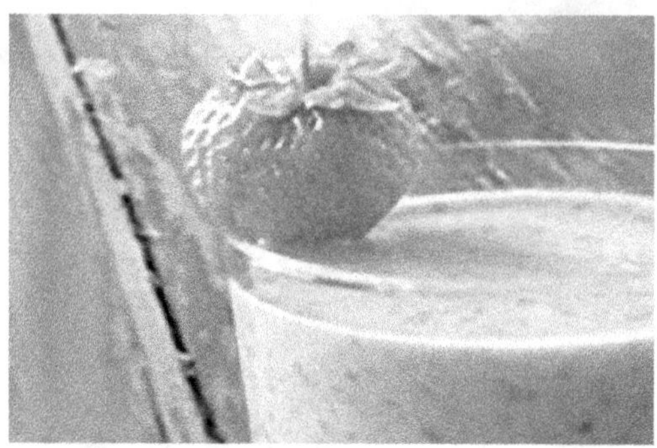

A6. Strawberry Date Surprise Smoothie

Serving size: makes 2 smoothies
Time to make: 10 minutes

Ingredients

2 cups fresh / or frozen strawberries
2 cups spinach washed and stalks removed
6 medjool dates / or 8 dried chopped dates
2 cups filtered water / or coconut water
1 tablespoon sacha inchi protein powder
2 tablespoons lucuma powder
1 teaspoon camu camu powder

Method

1. If using dried dates, let them soak a few minutes in some of the water.
2. Place spinach, dates and water into a blender.
3. Blitz until well processed.
4. Add strawberries, sacha inchi, lucuma and camu camu then blitz until well processed and smooth.
5. Pour into glasses and enjoy.

* Notes:

This is a vitamin C charged smoothie with no citrus fruit needed. Strawberries are high in vitamin C and camu camu is an extremely potent vitamin C berry. Lucuma contains beta-carotene to support the immune system making this smoothie a good marriage for fighting the flu.

Protein powder is an important element in smoothies, it helps carry the sugars to even out the glycaemic load. Protein supports our immune system, our metabolism and helps our bodies to sustain lean muscle.

NEXT Berry Smoothie recipe:
| A7 | Strawberry Fields Smoothie| Pg.14

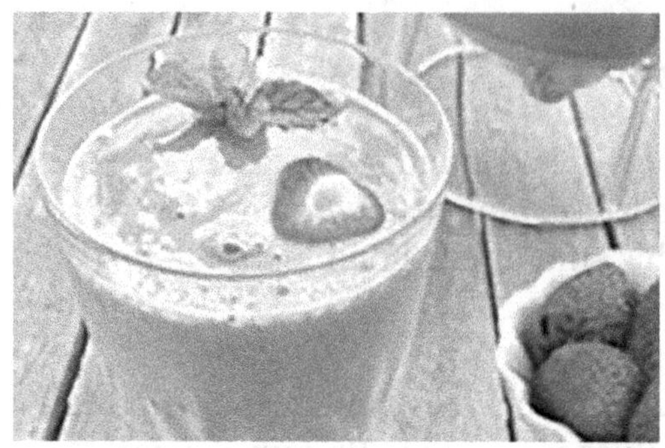

A7. Strawberry Fields Smoothie

Serving size: makes 2 smoothies
Time to make: 10 minutes

Ingredients

2 cups fresh / or frozen strawberries
2 frozen bananas, skin removed, chopped
2 large cups almond milk / or milk of your choice / or coconut water
2 teaspoons maqui berry powder / or acai berry powder
1 tablespoon maca powder
2 tablespoons lucuma powder

Method

1. Place all ingredients into a blender.
2. Blitz until all the fresh fruit is processed to a smooth texture.
3. Pour into glasses and enjoy.

* Notes:

Strawberries are a low calorie food high in vitamin C and manganese. They are a good detoxifier.

I love maca powder because it's not only delicious but it also supports the thyroid. However, maca powder is a product that a few people may react to.

If you are not used to maca powder, try using only a teaspoon at first, then increase it if you have no reaction. The usual reaction presents as minor stomach cramps. Most people have no problems at all, but I want you to be fully informed, just in case you are the exception.

NEXT: Section B | Green Smoothie recipes | Pg.17

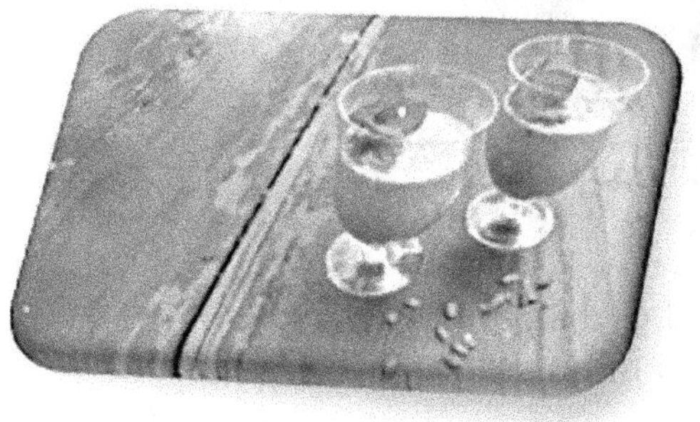

SECTION B

GREEN SMOOTHIE recipes

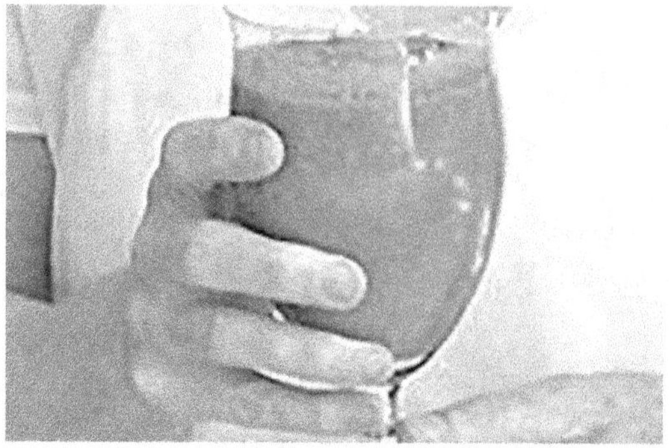

B1. Avocado Green Smoothie

Serving size: makes 2 smoothies
Time to make: 10 minutes

Ingredients

2 cups spinach / or silver beet
1 apple
1 ripe avocado
2 oranges skin removed / or 1 grapefruit
1 tablespoon liquid raw honey
1 lemon - juice only
1 handful of mint leaves / or parsley
2 cups filtered water / or coconut water
2 teaspoons maca powder
1 tablespoon sacha inchi protein powder
2 teaspoons naturally probiotic fermented greens powder (the green smoothie shot)

Method

1. Wash and tear spinach, remove tough stalks, then place in blender.

2. Chop apple, oranges and avocado into bite size pieces and place in blender.
3. Add honey and mint leaves / or parsley to blender.
4. Place 2 cups of water in blender and blitz all ingredients until well processed.
5. Add remaining maca powder, sacha inchi and fermented greens powder with the lemon juice - then blitz until smooth.

* Notes:

For those who don't like bananas but like a creamy texture, the avocado is the star. Not forgetting all the healthy plant based oils the avocado offers.

The green smoothie shot powder takes this smoothie up a notch; offering digestive enzymes and good bacteria so that optimum absorption is addressed.

NEXT Green Smoothie recipe:
| B2 | Berry Green Smoothie | Pg.20

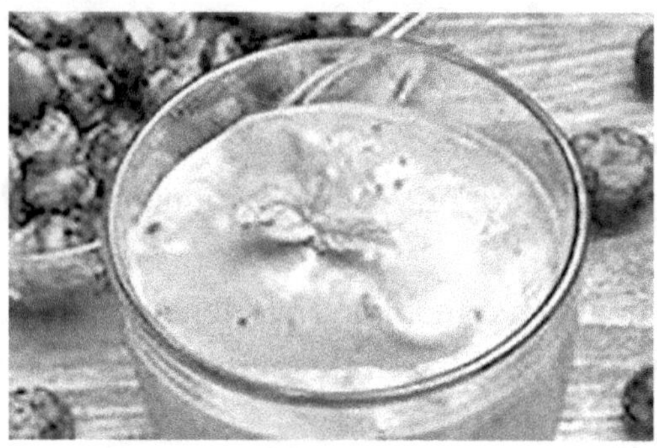

B2. Berry Green Smoothie

Serving size: makes 2 smoothies
Time to make: 10 minutes

Ingredients

2 cups spinach / or silver beet
1 apple
1 cup mixed fresh berries (strawberries, blueberries, blackberries)
1 banana (skin removed) chopped / fresh / or frozen
1 lemon - juice only
2 cups coconut water / or filtered water
2 tablespoons sacha inchi protein powder
1 tablespoon chia seeds
2 teaspoons maqui berry / or acai berry powder
2 teaspoons naturally probiotic fermented greens powder (the green smoothie shot)

Method

1. Wash and tear spinach, remove tough stalks, then place in blender.
2. Chop apple, discard core, then place in blender.
3. Add berries, banana, lemon juice and coconut water to blender

then blitz until well processed.

4. Add remaining ingredients, sacha inchi, chia seeds, maqui berry powder and green smoothie shot.
5. Blitz once more until well blended and smooth.

* Notes:

This smoothie has it all by adding the high antioxidant berries and berry powder. Maqui Berry is a good detoxifier.

A natural probiotic powder is my signature for a healthy smoothie as it contributes healthy bacteria to aid digestion and balance gut health.

NEXT Green Smoothie recipe:
| B3 | Citrus Green Smoothie | Pg.22

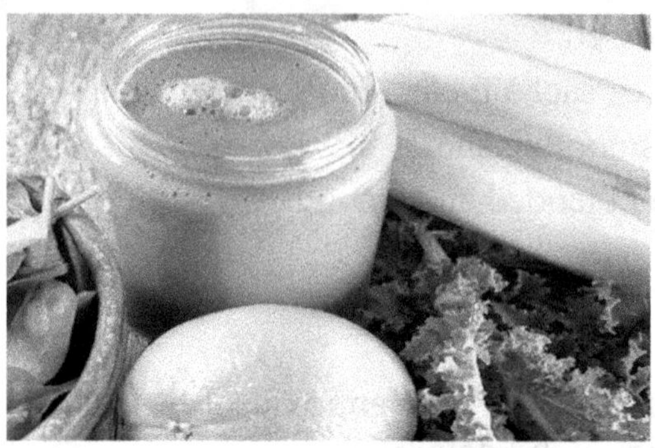

B3. Citrus Green Smoothie

Serving size: makes 2 smoothies
Time to make: 10 minutes

Ingredients

2 cups spinach / or silver beet
1 stalk of celery
2 bananas, fresh or frozen, skin removed
1 grapefruit / or large orange, skin removed
1 lemon - juice only
1 handful of mint leaves and / or a knob of fresh ginger
2 cups filtered water / or coconut water
2 tablespoons sacha inchi protein powder
1 tablespoon lucuma
2 teaspoons naturally probiotic fermented greens powder (the green smoothie shot)

Method

1. Wash and tear spinach, remove tough stalks, then place in blender with chopped celery and half the water, blitz until

well processed.

2. Add chopped grapefruit and bananas, then blitz again.
3. Add mint leaves and ginger to blender.
4. Place remaining water in blender and blitz all ingredients until well processed.
5. Add remaining dry ingredients with the lemon juice and blitz until smooth.

* Notes:

Citrus and mint are always good in a smoothie, because they are refreshing and uplifting.

A natural probiotic powder is my signature ingredient for a healthy green smoothie, as it contributes healthy bacteria to aid digestion and balance gut health.

NEXT Green Smoothie recipe:
| B4 | Cleansing Green Smoothie | Pg.24

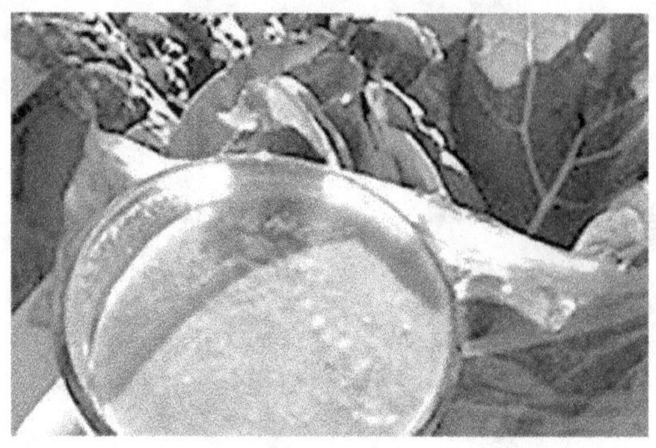

B4. Cleansing Green Smoothie

Serving size: makes 2 smoothies
Time to make: 10 minutes

Ingredients

2 cups spinach / or silver beet
1 cup cucumber
1 stalk celery
1 banana frozen
2 oranges
1 tablespoon liquid raw honey / or yacon syrup
1 knob fresh ginger
1 lemon - juice only
2 cups coconut water / or filtered water
1 tablespoon sacha inchi protein powder
1 tablespoon chia seeds
2 teaspoons naturally probiotic fermented greens powder (green smoothie shot)

Method

1. Wash and tear spinach. Remove tough stalks then place in the blender.

2. Chop celery, cucumber, oranges, ginger and banana then place in blender with half the water and blitz.
3. Add lemon juice, honey and remaining coconut water to blender then blitz until well processed.
4. Add remaining ingredients, sacha inchi, chia seeds and green smoothie shot.
5. Blitz once more until well blended and smooth.

* Notes:

This smoothie is the great cleanser. You can play around with the ingredient quantities to get the consistency that suits you.

A natural probiotic powder is my signature for a healthy green smoothie as it contributes healthy bacteria to aid digestion and balance gut health.

NEXT Green Smoothie recipe:
| B5 | Green Mango Smoothie | Pg.26

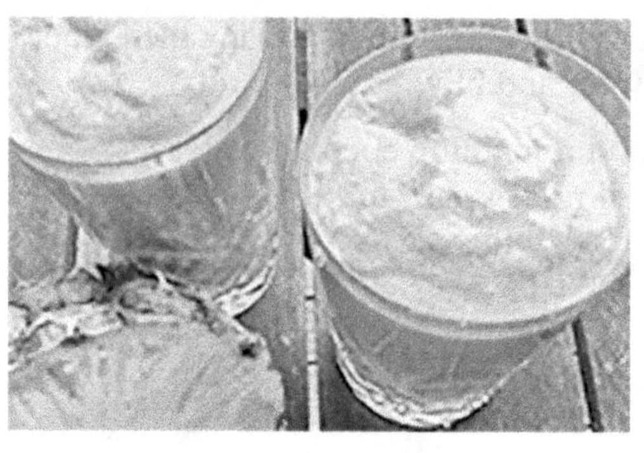

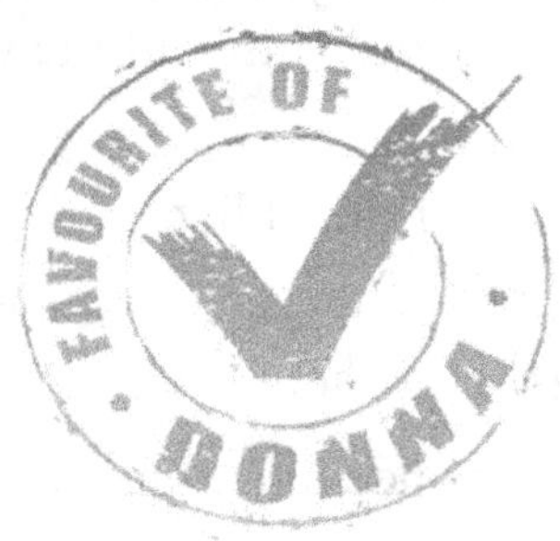

B5. Green Mango Smoothie

Serving size: makes 2 smoothies
Time to make: 10 minutes

Ingredients

2 cups spinach / or silver beet
1 mango
1 banana fresh / or frozen - skin removed
1 cup fresh diced pineapple
1 cup almond milk
1 cup coconut milk
1 tablespoon lucuma / or yacon powder
2 teaspoons naturally probiotic fermented greens powder (the green smoothie shot)

Method

1. Wash and tear spinach, remove tough stalks, then place in blender and blitz with some of the milk liquid.
2. Peel and dice mango then place in blender.
3. Place pineapple in blender.
4. Add coconut and almond milks to blender then blitz all ingredients until well processed.

5. Add the lucuma and fermented greens powder and blitz until smooth.

* Notes:

Mango and pineapple for me are decadent fruits, so delicious in taste and texture. Fortunately, fresh mangoes and pineapple are easier to find in New Zealand these days.

If you don't like coconut or almond milk, this smoothie is still a winner when it is made with filtered water or coconut water.

Mangoes have many health benefits, but here is one that I like. The antioxidant zeaxanthin, found in mangoes, filters out harmful blue light rays and is thought to play a protective role in eye health and help ward off damage from macular degeneration.

NEXT Green Smoothie recipe:
| B6 | Big Vit C Green Smoothie | Pg.28

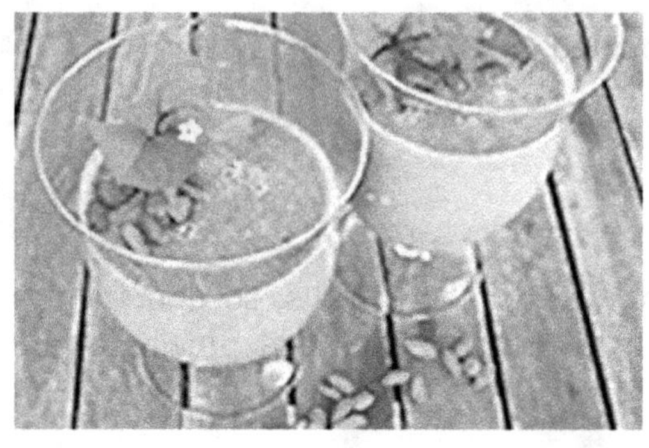

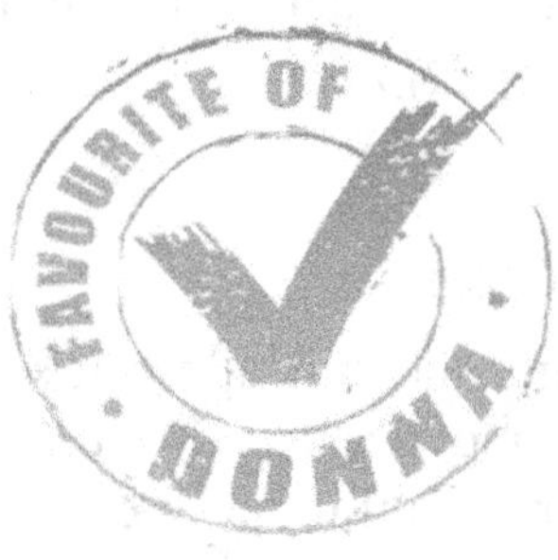

B6. Big Vit C Green Smoothie

Serving size: makes 2 smoothies
Time to make: 10 minutes

Ingredients

2 cups spinach or silver beet
1 apple skin on
1 banana fresh or frozen, skin removed
2 kiwi fruit, skin removed
1 knob fresh ginger, peeled
1 lemon - juice only
2 cups filtered water or coconut water
2 tablespoons sacha inchi protein powder
1 tablespoon chia seeds
1 tablespoon lucuma
1 teaspoon camu camu powder
2 teaspoons naturally probiotic fermented greens powder (the green smoothie shot)

Method

1. Wash and tear spinach remove tough stalks then place in blender and blitz with some of the water.

2. Chop the apple, banana and kiwi fruit into bite size pieces and put in blender.
3. Chop the ginger into fine pieces and add to blender.
4. Place remaining water in blender and blitz all ingredients until well processed.
5. Add remaining dry ingredients with the lemon juice and blitz until smooth.

* Notes:

I often like to make a green smoothie with a big vitamin C focus. Not just to keep the sniffles away but because a vitamin C charged smoothie always energises and uplifts me. It has a cleansing and renewing kick to it.

Apart from the vitamin C abundance in leafy greens, kiwifruit and lemon juice, it is the camu camu powder that is the star here. Camu camu has many more times Vitamin C than oranges.

A natural probiotic powder is my signature for a healthy green smoothie as it contributes healthy bacteria to aid digestion and balance gut health.

NEXT Green Smoothie recipe:
| B7 | Tropical Green Smoothie | Pg.30

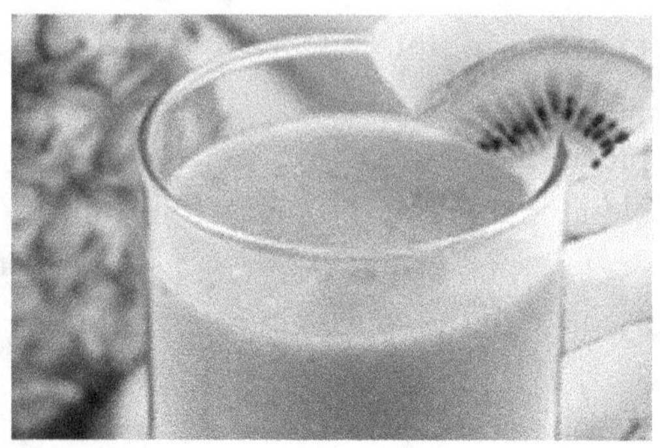

B7. Tropical Green Smoothie

Serving size: makes 2 smoothies
Time to make: 10 minutes

Ingredients

2 cups spinach / or silver beet
1 stalk of celery
1 orange - skin removed
1 cup fresh pineapple
1 banana fresh / or frozen skin removed
1 lemon - juice only
1 handful fresh mint leaves only
2 cups coconut water / or filtered water
2 tablespoons sacha inchi protein powder
1 tablespoon chia seeds
2 teaspoons maca powder
2 teaspoons naturally probiotic fermented greens powder (green smoothie shot)

Method

1. Wash and tear spinach, remove tough stalks then place in blender and blitz with some of the water.

2. Chop celery, orange, pineapple and banana then place in blender.
3. Add mint, lemon juice and remaining coconut water to blender and blitz until well processed.
4. Add remaining ingredients, sacha inchi, chia seeds, maca and green smoothie shot.
5. Blitz once more until well blended and smooth.

* Notes:

When peeling the orange be sure to leave some white pith between the orange peel and flesh. This pith contains just as much vitamin C as the orange flesh and has more fibre.

A natural probiotic powder is my signature for a healthy green smoothie as it contributes healthy bacteria to aid digestion and balance gut health.

NEXT: Section C | Decadent Smoothie recipes | Pg.33

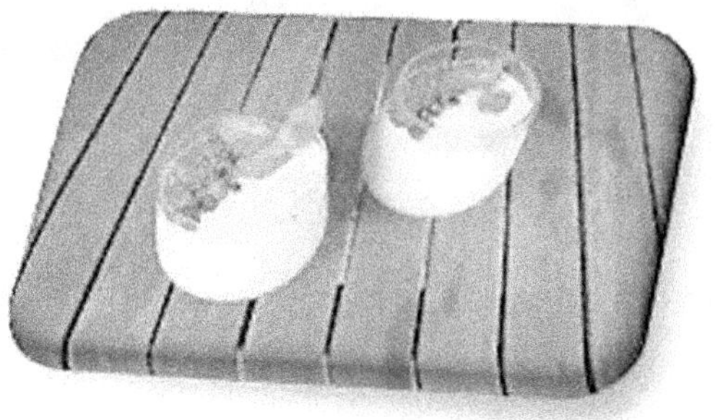

SECTION C

DECADENT SMOOTHIE recipes

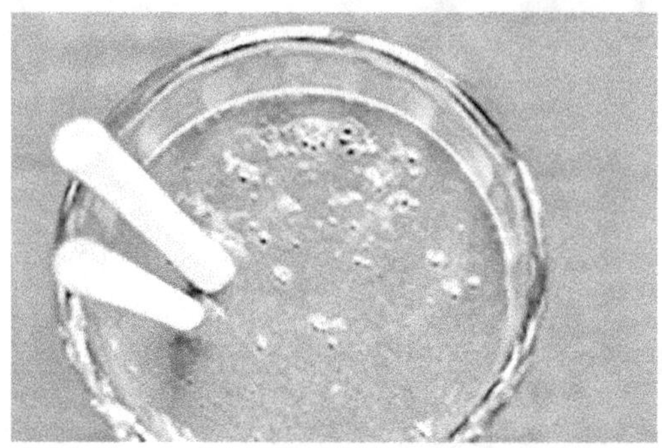

C1. Avocado Chocolate Decadence Smoothie

Serving size: makes 2 smoothies
Time to make: 10 minutes

Ingredients

2 frozen bananas, chopped, skin removed
1 avocado, peeled and diced, stone removed
2 tablespoons cacao powder
1 tablespoon lucuma / or yacon powder
2 cups almond milk / or milk of your choice
1 tablespoon maple syrup / or raw liquid honey
2 teaspoon naturally probiotic fermented greens powder

Method

1. Place all ingredients into a blender.
2. Blitz until banana is processed and a smooth texture appears.
3. Pour into glasses and enjoy.
4. Optional: roll truffles in maqui berry powder on a plate, to dust exterior of the truffles before refrigerating.

* Notes:

For those of you who are addicted to my chocolate mousse torte, this is your kind of smoothie.

NEXT Decadent Smoothie recipe:
| C2 | Chocolate Peanut Butter Lover Smoothie | Pg.36

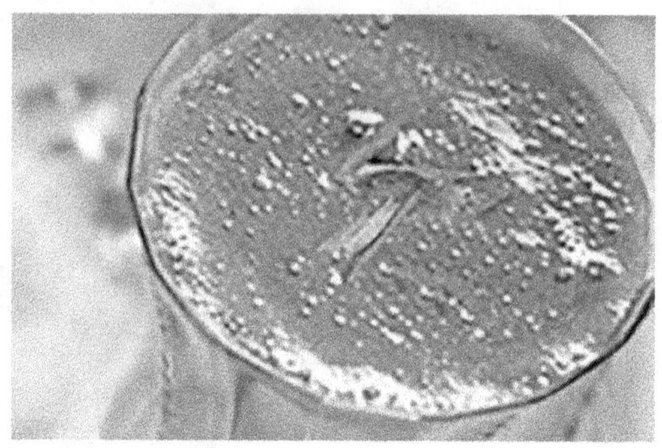

C2. Chocolate Peanut Butter Lover Smoothie

Serving size: makes 2 smoothies
Time to make: 5 minutes

Ingredients

2 frozen bananas - chopped and skin removed
2 tablespoons cacao powder
1 tablespoon cacao nibs
1 tablespoon of peanut butter
2 cups almond milk / or milk of your choice
1 tablespoon maple syrup / or raw liquid honey
1 dash of vanilla extract / or paste

Method

1. Place all ingredients into a blender.
2. Blitz until banana is processed and a smooth texture appears.
3. Pour into glasses and enjoy.

* Notes:

This chocolate peanut butter smoothie is perfect for recovering after a workout or hard day of physical work, you can add some sacha inchi protein powder, if you really want to have a protein fix. This is a really good smoothie for children after school.

NEXT Decadent Smoothie recipe:
| C3 | Quick Chocolate 'Pick-me-up' Smoothie | Pg.38

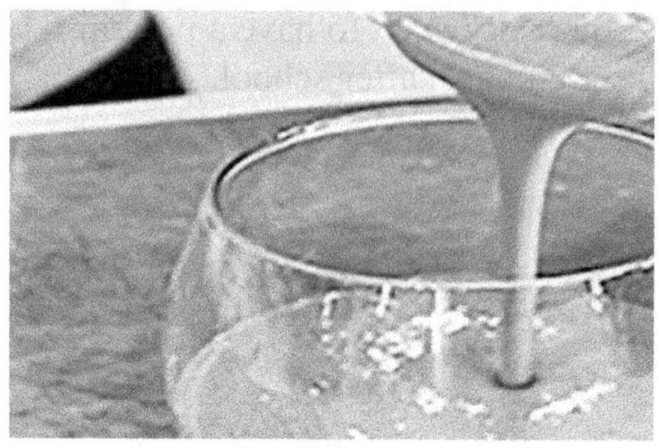

C3. Quick Chocolate Pick-me-up Smoothie

Serving size: makes 2 smoothies
Time to make: 5 minutes

Ingredients

2 frozen bananas, chopped, skin removed
2 tablespoons cacao powder
1 tablespoon of cacao nibs (if you don't have them, you can leave them out)
2 tablespoons cacao powder
2 tablespoons lucuma powder / or yacon powder
2 cups almond milk / or milk of your choice
1 tablespoon maple syrup / or raw liquid honey

Method

1. Place all ingredients into a blender.
2. Blitz until banana is processed and a fluffy smooth texture appears.
3. Pour into glasses and enjoy.

* Notes:

I love this smoothie in summertime late afternoon if I'm feeling a little low and I feel I can't make it to dinner. It is delicious, fast, easy, and slips down perfectly.

Cacao is a great mood elevator, so you will soon find yourself emerging from the doldrums.

NEXT Decadent Smoothie recipe:
| C4 | Feijoa Surprise Smoothie | Pg.40

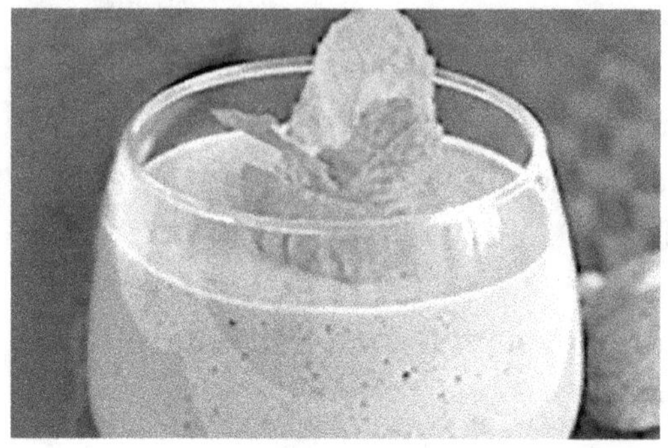

C4. Feijoa Surprise Smoothie

Serving size: makes 2 smoothies
Time to make: 10 minutes

Ingredients

2 frozen bananas, chopped, skin removed
2 feijoas, skinned and sliced
1 kiwi fruit
1 handful of chopped dried dates (soaked in a little water for 10 minutes)
1 handful of mint leaves
1 tablespoon sacha inch protein powder
1 tablespoon lucuma / or yacon powder
2 cups coconut water / or plain filtered water / or milk of your choice
2 teaspoons maca powder

Method

1. Place the soaking dates, bananas and some of the water into a blender and blitz.
2. Add remaining fruit with the remaining water and mint leaves then blitz until smooth.

3. Finally add the sacha inchi, lucuma, and maca powders - then blitz until well processed.
4. Pour into glasses and enjoy.

* Notes:

Like most Kiwi kids, I grew up with feijoas. I sat under hedges in the autumn eating as many as I could, after school. It wasn't until I travelled, that I found in many other countries feijoas have never been heard of (even by our Australian neighbours!)

Feijoas contain flavonoids and saponins, which are chemical compounds believed to be good for heart health and lowering cholesterol. Feijoas are high in Vitamin C and fibre.

NEXT Decadent Smoothie recipe:
| C5 | Mango Smoothie | Pg.42

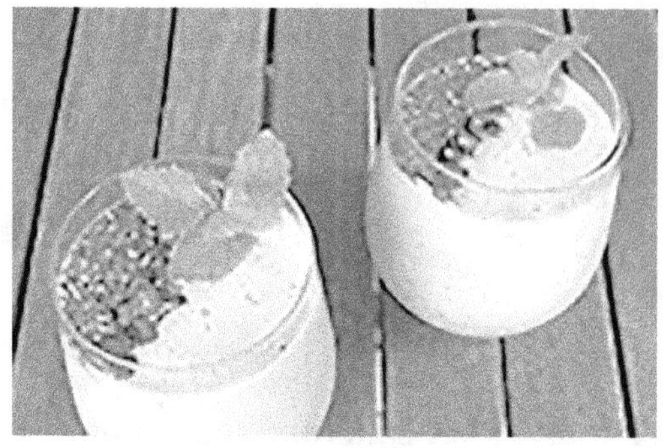

C5. Mango Smoothie

Serving size: makes 2 smoothies
Time to make: 10 minutes

Ingredients

2 frozen bananas, chopped, skin removed
1 mango, peeled and diced
2 oranges, peeled and diced
2 tablespoons lucuma powder / or yacon powder
1 teaspoon turmeric (optional)
1 cup coconut milk
1 cup almond milk
1 tablespoon raw liquid honey

Method

1. Place all ingredients into a blender.
2. Blitz until banana is processed and a fluffy smooth texture appears.
3. Pour into glasses and enjoy.

* Notes:

Mangoes are such a good all round fruit with many health benefits and plenty of fibre while being so decadently delicious. Turmeric goes well in this smoothie, and it also acts as an anti-inflammatory agent.

NEXT Decadent Smoothie recipe:
| C6 | Refreshing Decadence Smoothie | Pg.44

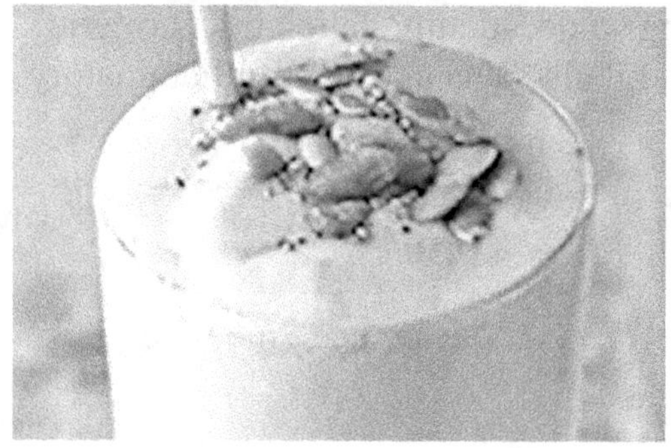

C6. Refreshing Decadence Smoothie

Serving size: makes 2 smoothies
Time to make: 10 minutes

Ingredients

2 frozen bananas, skin removed, chopped
1 mango
1 cup chopped pineapple
1 orange
1 handful of mint leaves
1 tablespoon sacha inch protein powder
1 tablespoon lucuma / or yacon powder
2 cups coconut water / or plain filtered water
1 tablespoon maple syrup / or raw liquid honey
2 teaspoons camu camu powder

Method

1. Place all ingredients into a blender.
2. Blitz until bananas are processed and a smooth texture appears.
3. Pour into glasses and enjoy.

* Notes:

A very refreshing and delicious smoothie that is high in vitamin C.

NEXT Decadent Smoothie recipe:
| C7 | Stone-fruit Indulgence Smoothie | Pg.46

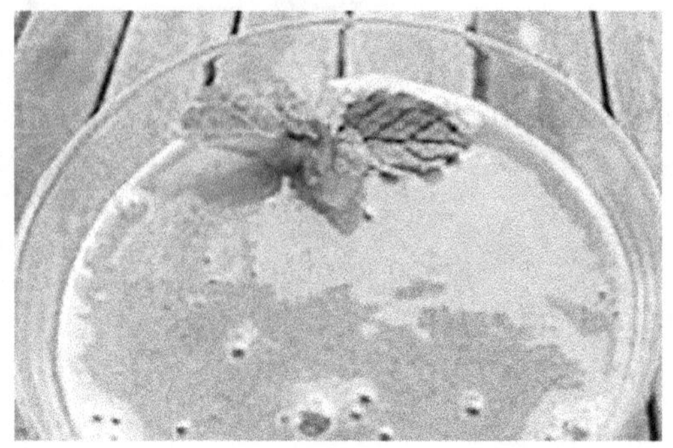

C7. Stone-fruit Indulgence Smoothie

Serving size: makes 2 smoothies
Time to make: 5 minutes

Ingredients

1 nectarine, de-stoned, chopped
2 frozen bananas, skin removed, chopped
1 peach - de-stoned and chopped
1 orange, skin removed, chopped
1 handful of chopped dried dates (soaked in a little water for 10 minutes)
1 handful of mint leaves
1 tablespoon sacha inch protein powder
1 tablespoon lucuma / or yacon powder
2 cups coconut water / or plain filtered water / or milk of your choice
2 teaspoons maca powder

Method

1. Place the soaking dates, bananas and some of the water into a blender and blitz.
2. Add remaining fruit with the remaining water and mint leaves then blitz until smooth.

3. Finally, add the sacha inchi, lucuma, and maca powders then blitz until well processed.
4. Pour into glasses and enjoy.

* Notes:

Stone fruit makes a lovely change and they are such a treat, when the season finally comes around.

NEXT: Health Benefits of Superfood Smoothies | Pg.48

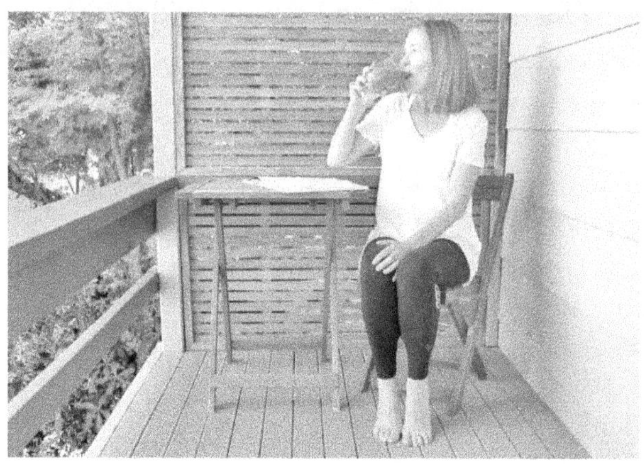

Top 10 Health Benefits of Superfood Smoothies

There are probably lots more, but here is *our* Top 10:

1. The blending process of smoothies helps to pre-digest food, which makes it easier for the digestive system to break down foods. This is extremely beneficial for those with already compromised digestive systems.

2. Equally, for athletes or those with high energy needs, the digestive system doesn't have to work so hard to make nutrition available. Thus conserving energy.

3. Many important vitamins and minerals are locked in the cellular walls of wholefood. The blending process helps rupture these walls so nutrients can be more easily released.

4. Fruit and vegetables in their whole form contain fibre. Fibre helps to promote gut function and peristalsis. Fibre can help control blood sugar levels.

   In people with diabetes, fibre— particularly soluble fibre — can slow the absorption of sugar and help improve blood sugar levels. A healthy diet that includes insoluble fibre may also reduce the risk of developing type 2 diabetes.

5. Smoothies are more substantial than juices and therefore I class them as more of a meal than a drink, they are thicker and more filling - as well as being more nutritionally balanced.

6. A smoothie containing fruit, vegetables and lean protein can help keep you feeling full for longer and boost your energy levels.

7. Smoothies are quick and easy to make, perfect for time poor situations and when sustenance is urgently needed.

8. Smoothies are ideal for sports recovery because they are easy to digest and instantly satisfying whilst returning depleted nutrients to muscles.

9. Apart from fruit and vegetables, you can add herbs, spices and superfoods to your smoothies to super boost the nutritional potency.

10. Lastly, making and drinking smoothies is a fun - not to mention 'delicious' - way to boost your health.

* * *

PHOTO Opposite left: Donna drinking her daily morning Green Smoothie on the deck.

Will Superfood Smoothies work for you?

Superfoods sceptics will say that there is no 'absolute proof' (yet) that putting all these good things into your body will lead to better health in the long-run. How do I answer that challenge? I say …

There's one way to know for *sure* ...

Try superfoods … then monitor the results for yourself! Superfoods obtained from a reputable source will be natural, nutrient-rich, and uncontaminated by chemicals and preservatives; unlike most of the foodstuffs you consume every day from your local supermarket. Trying them for a reasonable period of 2-3 months should reveal whether they will deliver the benefits that I and others claim to receive. This would be similar to your doctor trying a medication for a period to see if it works for you. However, if you have any concerns about taking superfoods you should get your doctor's 'go ahead' to try them, first.

Mainstream …

Mainstream medical professionals (apart from surgeons, physical therapists, and psychological counsellors) mainly seem to focus on drug-based *solutions* to health problems; and they usually come with a long list of potential 'side-effects' and legal disclaimers.

The bottom line of the small print boils down to the fact that 'you are choosing to take this drug at your own risk' and, having been warned, don't think you can sue the drug company if it all goes horribly wrong.

My Experience …

My experience (along with a wealth of anecdotal evidence) of superfoods is that I *feel* better, my brain seems to work better, and medical conditions, that I couldn't find an answer for using traditional medicine (drugs), went away.

Balance ...

Of course, you need to approach superfoods (like anything else) in a balanced and sensible way. So, if one superfood smoothie makes you feel better, don't drink ten of them! It won't be 10 times better for you. In fact, it would be bad for you. Just like abusing caffeine or alcohol. Or anything.

Common sense ...

Your body has natural tolerances and can only absorb certain amounts of anything each day. That's why many of the vitamins in supplement capsules are wasted and pass through your body without being absorbed. It is worth finding out how much of any vitamin or nutritional supplement your body needs per day and keeping track of your intake. It is not only safer, but it could save you flushing lots of money, literally, down the toilet.

Drugs v. Natural ...

As I get older, having experienced both sides of the equation in trying to keep my brain and body healthy, I prefer the natural approach in my daily life. It is working for me.

I believe, adding a daily nutrient-rich superfood smoothie to your diet will work for you too.

It might even change your life.

Donna Davidson

- November, 2016.

* * *

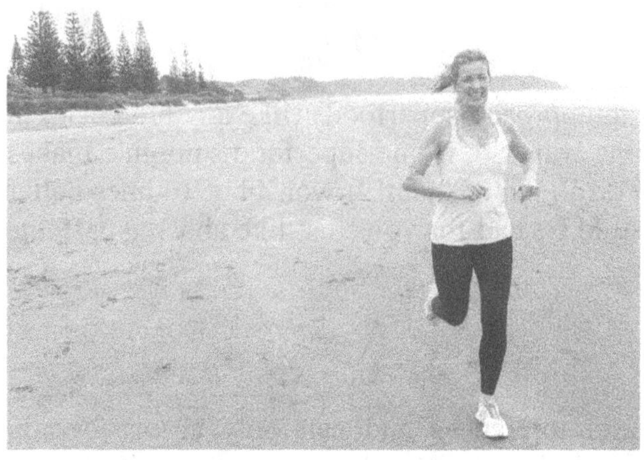

Donna Davidson Biography

- Author, business woman, recipe creator, 'superfoodie'.

Living happily by the Pacific Ocean, in New Zealand's beautiful North Island, Donna's primary passion has always been health, fitness and well-being.

Donna began her fitness career as an aerobics instructor; after receiving her diploma from Lords Gym in Perth, Australia, she trained at Jane Fonda's Workout Studio in Beverly Hills, California.

After establishing her own fitness studio back in Auckland, New Zealand, Donna was chosen to teach aerobics to New Zealand's Americas Cup yacht squad, as part of a new fitness and motivational program preparing them, for their first Americas Cup challenge.

Later, while working in the superfoods industry, Donna experienced the profound benefits of adding superfoods to her regular diet. She now credits superfoods with helping her conquer 2 major health challenges in her life; dangerously high blood pressure and 'cyclic vomiting' syndrome.

Donna also realized that she had much more energy, and increased mental acuity.

Wanting to *share* her discoveries with like-minded people, she decided to found her own superfoods company and online store; with the 'modest' aim of teaching as many people as possible about the benefits of superfoods, and making it easy for them to obtain them online.

The result was superfoodies.co.nz, which she created with the help of her friend, Kay Wood. Her goal was simple: to source the highest-quality superfood products and teach simple, sensible, delicious ways for ordinary folks to enjoy their health benefits - without any hype or exaggeration.

Donna's first book in Donna's 'health through nutrition' series, '21 Best Cacao (natural chocolate) Recipes' was launched in November, 2015, and quickly became an Amazon best seller - reaching the #1 spot several times! It's available in both Kindle and Print book formats on Amazon.

This is the second book, '21 Best Superfood Smoothies'. It gives you 21 delicious ways to easily drink yourself to better health. It's also available in both Kindle and Print book formats on Amazon.

Donna's third book, on 'Berry brain-foods' contains 21 of the best superfood berry recipes that help us slow the ageing process and retain mental sharpness, as we get older.

If you enjoyed this book, you'll definitely want to grab that one too. '21 Best Brain Food Berry Recipes' is available on Amazon in both Kindle eBook and Print book formats.

* * *

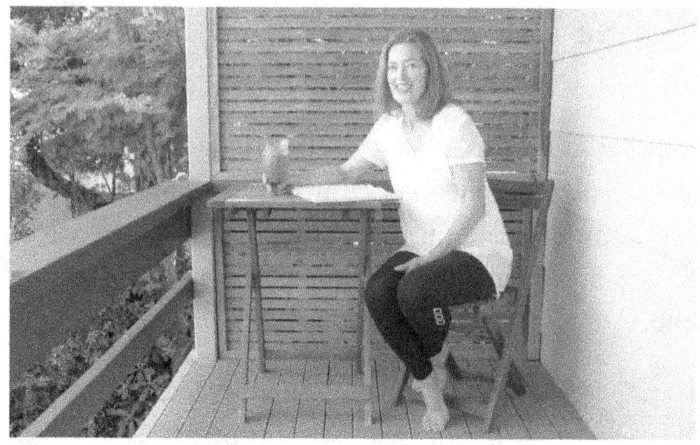

Donna's High Cholesterol story, in her own words...

"Despite a strong sporting background and regular fitness regime, I still battled debilitating health issues earlier in my life, for which I couldn't seem to find an answer.

Quite by accident, the answer came when I landed a job in the superfoods industry; I experienced increasingly positive changes by adding specific superfoods to my daily diet.

I had been diagnosed with 'cyclic vomiting' syndrome. On average, once a month I would throw up for 24 hours, which just wiped me out physically. When I started having a green smoothie every morning this cycle soon completely disappeared.

I realized that my daily green smoothie was alkalising my digestive system and setting me up for the day. A second (unexpected) consequence was the rapid reduction of my bad cholesterol.

I have always been very fit and slim, so I'd been totally shocked to find my cholesterol was at a dangerous level.

Although my mother had suffered from angina, and died with dangerously high cholesterol, aged 64, I had always considered myself 'fit and healthy' (despite my vomiting problem) and it had never occurred to me that I could be susceptible too.

After 3 months of drinking my green smoothie, my cholesterol went from 7.3 to 4.8. The result not only wowed *me*... but they *stunned* the nurse reading them out to me over the phone! I kept my printed test result sheets to prove to myself that I hadn't dreamt it, because even *I* couldn't believe it for ages. It took time to really sink in. I think, because it was literally life-changing for me.

To write the books in my 'Discover Superfoods' series I've had to draw deeply from all the knowledge I gained over 6 years of working in the superfoods industry; in order to create some of the best, easy-to-make, health-giving, superfood recipes available.

These recipes will help you add loads of wonderful superfoods to your normal diet, in ways that are not just super-nutritious and delicious, but often down-right decadent.

Please share your experiences with me, or ask me any questions you may have. I'd love to hear from you."

Donna Davidson

- November, 2016.

* * *

FOLLOW :: Donna on Facebook :: Facebook.com/SuperFoodies
EMAIL :: Donna :: info@superfoodies.co.nz

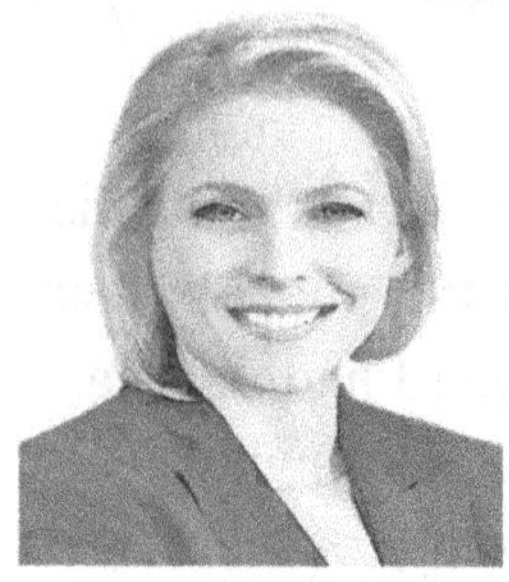

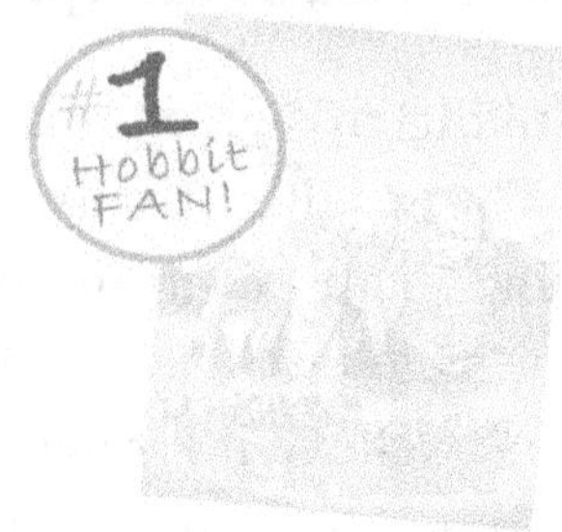

Kay Wood Biography

- Author, blogger, copywriter, web marketer, ‘superfoodie’.

Originally from the world of advertising and marketing, Kay has more recently specialised in copywriting and content creation for the Internet. She also adores anything Tolkien, especially Hobbits.

For nearly 10 years Kay has been 'ghost-writing' info blogs for online businesses and offering her help to clients struggling to turn their awkward prose and bad spelling into simple and easily understood information about their products and services.

Kay and Donna became friends while working together to create Donna's superfoodies.co.nz website, in late 2013. Kay also worked closely with Donna to help her realise her ideas for the 'look and feel' of her superfood product packaging and the ‘Superfoodies’ logo design.

Kay and Donna found themselves ‘clicking’ as a team during that creative process. They both shared a common desire to present in an honest and balanced way the genuine health benefits to be gained by incorporating superfoods into one's diet - while at the same time dialling back some of the hype surrounding superfoods.

Kay’s story, in her own words ...

“When I suggested to Donna that putting together some of her favourite and most delicious superfood recipes into a cookbook 'might be a good idea', to help show people how many ways superfoods can be incorporated into their diet, she initially hesitated because it sounded like such a daunting prospect to cover all, or even most, of the major superfoods in one book.

I later modified the original idea, suggesting to Donna that she should create a series of short, practical recipe books sharply focused on only one superfood in each book, pared down to the 21 absolute best recipes that Donna could come up with.

We both agreed that cacao would be the perfect superfood for book #1 - because everyone loves chocolate right? And healthy, or certainly healthier, ways to enjoy chocolate have got to be a great addition to any chocolate lover's recipe book collection.

So, with me cracking the whip and Donna creating, making, baking, eating and perfecting the recipes, our first modest little book, 'Discover Superfoods #1: 21 Best Cacao Recipes' was born. If you haven't got it yet, and you love chocolate, I can really recommend it (as a chocoholic myself!) Once you have, I'm sure you'll love the wonderful cacao (natural organic chocolate) recipes as much as we do!

Thanks for buying this book of healthy smoothie recipes, too! You won't regret it. Drinking one superfood smoothie every morning, you can literally drink your way to better health. Try creating your own unique variations around Donna's base recipes, using the 'Recipe Diary' in the back of this book. (See pg.88) You can have fun while learning what combinations work best for you.

If you enjoy Donna's recipes, please give us a nice review on Amazon, because that will really help us spread the good word about superfoods to those who still haven't heard that healthy, natural alternatives to junk food actually exist!"

Kay Wood - November, 2016.

Living in Aotearoa / New Zealand / Middle Earth - with the Hobbits.

What are Superfoods?

Superfoods are a special category of foods found in nature: these foods are superior sources of the essential nutrients and antioxidants that our bodies need, but cannot make themselves.

Superfoods are calorie-sparse and nutrient-dense, so they pack a lot of punch for their weight and deliver more of what our bodies need in one go. Foods that have been elevated to superfood status in recent years include those rich in antioxidants, vitamins, minerals, essential fatty acids, including omega-3 fatty acids.

Contrary to what some people wrongly believe, Superfoods are NOT nutrition created through advancements in food sciences. They are actually looking back to nature for what it does best: providing us with amazing and complex combinations of nutrients, beautifully balanced to supply us with what our bodies require to flourish.

This is simply going back to the wild and harnessing foods in their natural forms, with all their benefits intact. It is celebrating nature's wealth of nutrients in all its varieties. We have within our reach a true powerhouse of natural ingredients to provide us with the nutrition we need for healthy living.

Many superfoods are unique to their own geographical position in the world and this is usually because their local environment was perfect for producing them. Fortunately, in our modern world of advanced communication, travel and cultural appreciation, we are currently discovering an abundance of nutrient-rich superfoods we have previously never heard of. e.g. superfoods from South America, like the sacha inchi seeds, maqui berries, maca root, lucuma, and camu camu.

See Superfood Descriptions on pg.60 of this book, for more info.

There is no official definition of a superfood, and the EU has banned the use of the word on packaging, but that hasn't stopped many food brands from funding academics to research the health benefits of their products. Nor does it deter the health conscious from seeking and following eating regimes abundant with good nutrient-dense foods that they enjoy and feel the benefits of.

Superfoods can be processed under 40 degrees Celsius without damaging their nutritional profile and being classed as 'raw foods'. This makes storage and availability more convenient and versatile. e.g. superfood powders for smoothies and snacks are generally dried below 40 degrees Celsius.

An awareness of the kinds of foods that we're now calling 'superfoods', has been increasing rapidly over the last few years. Along with a better appreciation for how the foods we consume affect our bodies, as well as our long-term health.

We're also finding ourselves being 're-introduced' to many of the foods that were well-known to past generations, yet have been neglected for decades. We have lost touch with the knowledge of plants and natural compounds that our supposedly more primitive ancestors used to survive and heal themselves, before drugs were invented.

This is a knowledge that we all need to re-discover – if only to balance out the modern reliance on artificial drug based treatments. We're not saying that all drugs are bad, but returning to a lot of the effective yet natural ways of maintaining and restoring our health can't be a bad thing, either.

That way we can save drugs for serious health problems that require sudden, dramatic intervention. Thus, we may actually increase their efficacy and, by reducing their usage, also reduce the risk of creating drug resistant bacteria and the instances of harmful side-effects. Our immune systems will also thank us. Drugs often weaken our immune systems by killing the pro-biotic bacteria in our gut, interfering with the body's ability to digest food properly.

* * *

Superfoods Descriptions + Info

These are the dried superfoods Donna uses in her recipes:

Sacha Inchi protein powder: Vegetable protein powder from the South American Sacha Inchi seed. Contains 60% complete protein, all essential amino acids, as well as the omega essential fatty acids. Easily digestible and light nutty flavour. Perfect for pre/post workout smoothies, to maintain and build muscle.

More about Sacha Inchi powder + where to buy it :
Type into your web browser: www.superfoodies.co.nz/des-a

Maqui Berry powder: Reported to have the highest antioxidant/anthocyanin content than any other fruit or berry. Grows wild in the patagonian rain forests of Chile and Argentina. Contributes to cardiovascular health, cellular protection against oxidative stress, immune support and detoxification. Maqui berry powder is deep purple in colour and has a delicious rich berry flavour.

More about Maqui Berry powder + where to buy it :
Type into your web browser: www.superfoodies.co.nz/des-b

Acai Berry powder: Like maqui berry powder, acai has a very high antioxidant content with unique structures of anthocyanins for cellular protection and phytochemicals believed to lower cholesterol levels. Contains high levels of vitamin E and essential fatty acids to support clear smooth skin. Acai is low in sugar, deep purple in colour and perfect for smoothies and breakfast recipes.

More about Acai Berry powder + where to buy it :
Type into your web browser: www.superfoodies.co.nz/des-c

Lucuma powder: Comes from a fruit native to the Peruvian Andean region. It provides beta-carotene known for immune support as well as calcium phosphorous and iron for energy. It has a low glycaemic score of around 25 while it imparts a natural sweet, creamy, citrusy, maple flavour.

More about Lucuma powder + where to buy it :
Type into your web browser: www.superfoodies.co.nz/des-d

Maca powder: Contains unique alkaloids known to stimulate the hypothalamus and pituitary glands which in turn improve the overall functioning of the endocrine system responsible for balancing hormones. Grown in Bolivia and Peru it has a vanilla/nutty taste which is very appealing in smoothies. Although one of the most popular and consumed superfoods it is a food that can make some people feel queasy or have stomach cramps, but this is not common. I recommend small doses to start with e.g. 1 teaspoon in a smoothie, working up to 1 tablespoon per day.

More about Maca powder + where to buy it :
Type into your web browser: www.superfoodies.co.nz/des-e

Yacon powder: A natural sweetener containing high levels of inulin a fructooligosaccharide that provides sweetness in a form that is indigestible by humans so they do not affect blood sugar levels and simply pass through the digestive tract to be eliminated. Since these sugars are not digested and also low in calories they are suitable for use in diet and low calorie foods.

More about Yacon powder + where to buy it :
Type into your web browser: www.superfoodies.co.nz/des-f

Yacon syrup: The same as yacon powder, it's GI is only ONE. I find this syrup delicious in recipes, cacao drinks and smoothies. It is the perfect substitute for maple syrup if you are watching your sugar intake, often not easy to find and unfortunately a little more expensive.

More about Yacon syrup + where to buy it :
Type into your web browser: www.superfoodies.co.nz/des-g

Camu Camu berry powder: The camu camu berry from the Amazon region is presenting higher levels of vitamin C than any other fruit tested to date. Latest results are showing 56 times more vitamin C than Lemons. It is a potent addition for any smoothie.

More about Camu Camu berry powder + where to buy it :
Type into your web browser: www.superfoodies.co.nz/des-h

Blueberry powder: Well known for its antioxidants and anthocyanins. It also contains resveratrol also found in grapes which has been linked to heart health. A convenient powder to add flavour to smoothies.

More about Blueberry powder + where to buy it :
Type into your web browser: www.superfoodies.co.nz/des-i

Chia seeds: A must have ingredient for a superfood pantry. When added to smoothies they make you feel full and satisfied for longer periods.Chia seeds contain more omega 3 fatty acids than salmon. They are low glycaemic and are another source of protein.

More about Chia seeds + where to buy it :
Type into your web browser: www.superfoodies.co.nz/des-j

Fermented greens powder: A powerful formula which acts as a natural probiotic because of the good bacteria produced from the fermentation process. This natural probiotic aids digestion, assists absorption and has many healing functions. It is my personal MUST HAVE in a morning smoothie to set me up for the day.

More about Fermented greens powder + where to buy it :
Type into your web browser: www.superfoodies.co.nz/des-k

Cacao powder: Cacao powder has an extremely high antioxidant score on the ORAC scale. By eating high antioxidant foods in our diet it is believed we are helping to guard against cellular and tissue damage which often lead to serious illness.

Magnesium is abundant in Cacao Powder and it is magnesium that is known to be the most important mineral for a healthy heart. Cacao is a mood elevator due to the presence of serotonin.

More about Cacao powder + where to buy it :
Type into your web browser: www.superfoodies.co.nz/des-l

Cacao butter: Is the ingredient that sets chocolate and other chocolate treats. It contains oleic acid which is the same healthy fat found in olive oil. It also is a good source of vitamin E. It does not need to be stored in the refrigerator. It melts to liquid at 35 degrees Celsius.

More about Cacao butter + where to buy it :
Type into your web browser: www.superfoodies.co.nz/des-m

Cacao nibs: Has a similar nutritional profile to cacao powder. Nibs are the shavings and fragments from the cacao bean. They add crunch and texture to chocolate treats and smoothies.

More about Cacao nibs + where to buy it :
Type into your web browser: www.superfoodies.co.nz/des-n

* * *

Superfoods Testimonials

These are a few typical examples of unsolicited testimonials and comments about superfood products from happy customers who purchased from Donna's own website: superfoodies.co.nz

Lost over 7kg and feeling so much better …

"Thank you so much for the healthy delicious treats for Christmas. I am still enjoying my new eating regime with super foods. I have lost over 7kg and feeling so much better in myself. Everyone comments on how well I look and that my skin is glowing. Coming along to your sugar free cooking class was the best thing I have done in a long time." **- Kate.**

* * *

My husband is really noticing the benefits …

"Nick my husband has been using the green smoothie powder and really noticing the benefits – he is a landscaper so needs the energy - plus he has sinus problems and this has really helped with that as well. Brilliant." **- Annemarie.**

* * *

Helping me cope with the stresses of my current life …

"Still going strong with the smoothies and have one most days. Really like them and I think they are helping me cope with the stresses of my current life – very sick husband, work, coping with ten staff, visitors and the rest of the daily grind. They fill me up now that I add soy or almond milk until the next meal and I have found that my sweet tooth has dissipated to a large degree – not wanting something sweet every day, which is a real bonus. So all good, and all thanks to you!" **- Sigrid.**

* * *

I'm 'regular as clock-work' – without medication … wahoo!

"I'm pleased to tell you that I am having a smoothie every morning and my Green Smoothie Shot and the great thing is, I have been able to stop taking the Laxsol tablets that I have had to take for years. I decided to stop taking them straight away because they aren't life threatening (just uncomfortable if it didn't work) to see if the Chia seeds and Green Smoothie Shot made any difference immediately and I'm pleased to say it has, and I've never been able to go off these tablets before, so now I'm 'regular as clock-work' and without medication … wahoo!

Now for the extra good news, **I have lost 2kgs in just under 2 weeks** of using the Chia Seeds, Cacao Powder and Green Smoothie Shot - so the products are obviously cleansing my body well. I'm using all natural 100% pure coconut water in my smoothies and a frozen banana which is awesome." – **Michele.**

* * *

Immediately noticed an increase in my energy and general wellbeing …

"At last I can get a fermented probiotic greens powder (Donna's Green Smoothie Shot) in New Zealand! I have been searching high and low for a fermented greens powder in New Zealand since I moved here some years ago. When living in Sydney I was introduced to this product and I immediately noticed an increase in energy and general wellbeing – I was overworked and I truly think that this is what helped keep me going. When I left Australia I took as much with me as I could carry in my case, but that is long gone and I have been missing it ever since.

So thank you 'SuperFoodies.co.nz' for bringing this wonderful product to New Zealanders – it is every bit as good as I remember!" – **Xenia.**

* * *

I have already made <u>double-lot</u> of Choc Fudge protein bars …

“Thank you very much for yesterday, I so enjoyed it. Have already made ‘double-lot’ of Choc Fudge protein bars and my children like them!” – **Hiria Wallace.**

* * *

Enhanced our well-being and energy (and didn’t get sick) …

“My husband and I have just returned from a month’s trip around Morocco and every morning we took “Green Smoothie Shot” without fail. We were pleasantly surprised we did not experience any sickness and felt this product enhanced our well-being and energy to make the most of our holiday.” – **Yvonne Porter.**

* * *

I learnt so much and changed my eating already …

“I learnt so much and have changed a few things with my eating already. Would love to carry on learning more.” – **Jodeen Mitchell.**

* * *

You are so passionate about healthy food …

“Thanks ladies! You’re both awesome. Very inspiring, as you are both so passionate about healthy food. Will try recipes out on my family – **Jeanette Pleijte.**

* * *

Read more Testimonials
superfoodies.co.nz/category/testimonials/

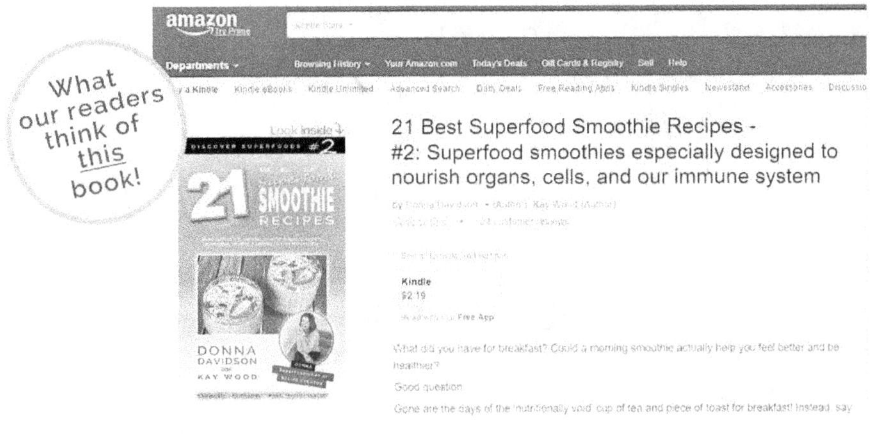

 5 Star Amazon Book Reviews:

- "Easy to follow recipes - excellent, especially for a smoothie newbie."
- "I couldn't wait for this book to come out on Amazon. I am a smoothie lover and strong believer in the health benefits of the [superfoods] powders."
- "This book is great for expanding my smoothie repertoire.
- "The recipes are delicious... more importantly, they make me feel great."
- "This book prompts me to try different and delicious combinations in my morning smoothie! Another amazing healthy recipe book from Donna!"
- "My kids LOVE them! Mom tested, Kid Approved!"
- "As a person with food sensitivities, I've found solace in vibrant, multi-ingredient smoothies. A book like this does a lot for a person like me."

See more reviews here > www.amazon.com/dp/B01J73OAKG

WHERE TO START?

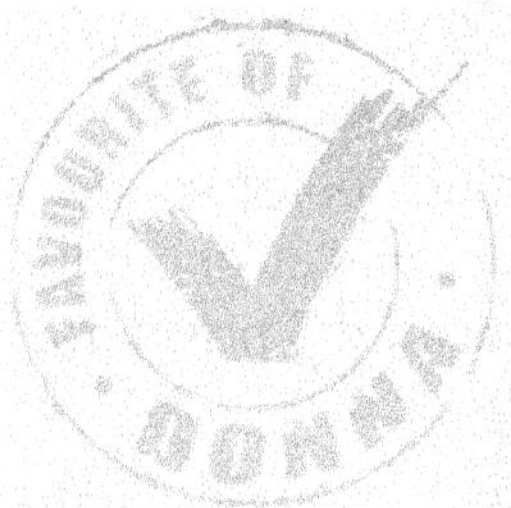

TRY ME!

Isn't 'fresh' always best?

And other Frequently Asked Questions, like:

1. What are all these superfood powders and dried processed products?
2. Isn't fresh always best?
3. What makes them 'super' foods - as opposed to ordinary foods?
4. How do these dried processed superfoods compare with fresh foods that are also called superfoods?
5. Are all these powders and dried stuff really superfoods?
6. Where can I get all these fancy dried superfood products?
7. Do they sell them in my local supermarket or do I have to go to a Health Food Shop?

* * *

If *you've* asked any of these questions, here are the answers, according to Donna and Kay:

QUESTION: "So, why are you using 'dried' superfood powders and products in these recipes?"

KAY'S ANSWER: This is something that often seems weird to people unfamiliar with using the dried forms of superfood products that are now available on the market.

In an ideal world, we would all have acai berries, maqui berries, blueberries, bananas, and cacao growing fresh in our backyards and we would pick them at the height of their potency and use them fresh every day.

Sadly, no matter where you live, this would be practically impossible. Either for climatic reasons, soil suitability, time poverty, lack of backyard garden space, lack of knowledge about how to actually grow and maintain these kinds of plants, and a zillion more reasons.

Even the supposedly 'fresh' fruits and vegetables we have available locally vary in nutritional value and taste, because of rising population numbers, they have to be grown quickly, picked, preserved, transported, displayed, and sometimes artificially enhanced to look appealing to consumers. The average 'fresh' tomato that most modern city dwellers eat is vastly different to the 'fresh' tomato that our grandparents or great-grandparents would have eaten. I remember my father growing tomatoes and strawberries in our small town New Zealand backyard and how 'gobsmack-ingly' delicious they were compared with the bland equivalents I purchase from the supermarkets these days.

When the population of the planet was relatively small, a mere 200 years ago, it was possible (at least theoretically) to grow enough food for the whole population of the world on the fertile farmland available, while also allowing enough time for excess land to lay 'fallow' for several years in order for the soil to recover the nutrients sucked out of it by the plants as they grew. That goodness, of course, was transferred to us when we ate those plants. Now, however, with farmland diminishing worldwide and poor farm and land management practices being common in many parts of the world, we already have less farmland available than is required to feed us all. This means that the land is being over utilised, the nutrients being stripped and never replaced, leading to less and less nutrients in the actual fruit and vegetables being grown on that land.

And then there's contamination from chemicals, such as fertilisers and pesticides, pollution, climate change, contamination from poor storage, unhealthy additives, and bad practices engaged in by unethical companies quite happy to put profit before their customers' health.

In an ideal world, 'fresh' would reign supreme. But in the real world, often the best we can do is combine 'fresh' (hopefully from the least contaminated sources) with high-quality dried nutrient sources - like the superfoods we recommend - in order to give our bodies and immune systems access to nutrients that aren't guaranteed to be in our food anymore.

If you live in a city, and especially if you have a busy, pressurised lifestyle, you probably don't have a garden, or the time to maintain one. My dad knew what nutrients his tomatoes needed and what kind of things were bad for them. Even though I ate his produce with glee, I never acquired his knowledge or skills and have never had much of a garden, sadly. Now, I wish I'd taken more notice and been more willing to learn from him.

I'm sure the same is true for many people, especially those younger than me; the whole idea of growing things yourself is a foreign concept. For some people even the idea of eating green things is foreign, and they think all food comes in packages that you heat up in a microwave. For those people, on a practical level, it would be much easier to throw some dried superfood ingredients into a blender, chop up a few available fruits or vegetables from the supermarket, and blend them all into a delicious smoothie in a couple of minutes, than to contemplate actually growing anything – never-mind having the land, plants or seeds, tools, fertilisers, knowledge and time to actually do it. Not to mention controlling pests, without risk to you, or the soil. Whoops, I mentioned it!

Is a tropical rainforest growing outside your window?

Many of the wonderful dried superfoods we use are only found in South America - probably because of the peculiarities of that climate and the evolution that occurred there in the isolation of the fertile tropical jungles. We think that buying superfoods from ethically responsible companies - who pick them 'fresh' at exactly the right moment, dry process them within an hour or two of being picked to lock in their nutrient content at its most potent - is a great way to access the tremendous nutrient value they contain.

Some still say, "You can get *everything* you need by eating fresh fruit and vegetables from the supermarket". If you read everything I wrote prior to this, and still believe that's a true statement, then you are entitled to your opinion. Donna and I would respectfully disagree with you. We have seen many people restore their health and well-being, as well as supporting their immune systems to fight and often eliminate stubborn health conditions. This is anecdotal evidence for sure, but, often, anecdotal evidence is only evidence waiting for science to catch up.

We can't guarantee that everybody who tries superfoods will experience the same results, but the same would be true if you visited the doctor and he recommended a course of treatment or certain medications. A doctor will never guarantee you anything. Also, try contacting the drug companies and see if they'll guarantee you that their products will work. Even the ones that have been supposedly approved and double-blind tested.

At the end of the day, as Donna and I often say, the 'proof is in the pudding' and you need to try something for a reasonable period of time and see if it works for you. Of course, you should do your 'due diligence'. Do as much research as you can, reference as much expert opinion as you can, try and find as much testimonial from those who have similar conditions to yourself and see what results they obtained, and then … you still end up with having to decide whether you will try them to see if they'll work for you.

This would be true of *anything*.

When Donna first tried green smoothies to see if they would help lower her high-cholesterol levels, a few years ago, she never expected them to eliminate her chronic 'cyclic vomiting' problem as well. That was a total surprise. Her life changed completely just because she added a green superfood smoothie every morning! There was no medical solution available at the time. The best she could do was to 'manage' the problem with injections of drugs.

My own experience is less dramatic: I was experiencing stomach pains and just feeling generally fatigued and unwell. When Donna sent me some 'green smoothie shot powder' which I added to a morning smoothie I came right within a week and have felt more balanced and that my stomach and digestion was working as it should. I don't feel queasy and nervous about my gut the way I previously did when it felt unstable and uncomfortable on a regular basis, despite the fact that my diet was comparatively healthy.

I hope my thoughts on the 'why' part of the "*why* do you use these kind of dried products?' question, has helped.

I'll let Donna explain her ideas of the pros and cons between 'fresh versus dried' superfoods, since she has much more expertise, not to mention experience, than me.

Kay Wood - November, 2016.

* * *

'Fresh' vs. 'Dried' Superfoods …

QUESTION: "How do these dried, processed superfoods compare with fresh foods that are also called 'superfoods'?"

DONNA'S ANSWER: I personally believe in and work with both.

When I'm time poor, I'm grateful to have my stash of dried superfoods in my pantry, so that I can whisk up a delicious and satisfying smoothie and be on my way to take on the day. When I have time to spare and have been fresh produce shopping I enjoy experimenting with produce in season mixed with my superfoods.

I know I can 'bank' on the variety of tastes and nutrition in dried superfoods, and they are as easy as having the stock in my pantry.

Fresh produce is not always at your fingertips, unless you have a prolific garden ... lucky you. So I say, you can 'have it all' by combining the use of dried and fresh (whatever's seasonally available).

Here are some 'Pros and Cons' - for fresh versus dried superfoods:

Fresh is Best - when:

1. You know you are buying or gardening organically.

2. Your produce is harvested at its peak nutritional stage.
3. Your produce is stored in a cool place or refrigerator.

Downside of 'Fresh':

1. Using fresh produce requires lots of your 'TIME' for organisation, storage, planning, and preparation.
2. Seasonal unavailability of your favourites.

Dried is Best - when:

1. They are harvested at their nutritional peak and immediately processed to lock in their nutritional profile.
2. You can safely buy organic and see where the product is from on the label.
3. Storage is more convenient and takes up less space.
4. No produce preparation in the form of cutting, washing etc.
5. Less shopping.
6. Less planning ahead.
7. If you buy from a reputable company, quality and purity is more certain.

Downside of 'Dried':

1. Taste is the only real downside to dried superfoods.

The huge advantage of dried superfoods is that they are preserved at the highest level of nutrient potency and degrade very slowly when well stored. But they can't beat the wonderful fresh 'taste' of local seasonal produce.

'Fresh' is delicious and nutritious; offering a wide variety of taste and flavour combinations, depending on the season. Whenever I make a smoothie or design a recipe I never rely solely on the dried superfood products because, although they may be delivering the desired nutritional punch that our bodies and immune systems need so desperately, our taste buds also need to enjoy themselves!

That's why my recipes are full of 'real foods' and 'superfoods', in the forms of fresh fruits, nuts, seeds, and vegetables, as well as dried superfoods. I want the recipes to be a balance between taste and health, so they deliver on both fronts. In previous generations we often believed that if it was good for you it had to 'taste bad' - but these days we expect healthy food to be delicious and delightful to our taste buds, as well.

That's my goal when I sit down to design any new recipe. If I'm modifying an existing recipe, it will be because I can improve either the nutritional content, or the taste factor, or both. That was pretty easy for this book because it's all about smoothie recipes so they weren't too hard to make delicious, or healthy either - as long as you only use quality ingredients. Please make sure you stick closely to my recipes and resist temptation to add any 'nasties', like extra sugar - or you'll undermine all my good work!

Sometimes, when you're beginning to add superfoods to your diet, your taste buds will need a little time to adjust to the lack of excess sugar and salt and other nasties that your system has been used to. Don't worry, after a very short time you will begin to enjoy the wonderful variety of natural flavours that were masked by these unhealthy additives in the past. *Then* your taste buds will begin to take you on a voyage of (re)discovery of flavours and taste sensations that you've been missing out on, or not enjoying to their fullest intensity.

Donna

- November, 2016.

* * *

Where can I get these dried superfoods?

If you haven't heard of some of the superfoods (fresh or dried) – like lucuma powder or acai berries, for example - that Donna uses in her recipes, you may be wondering, "Where may I obtain these weird and wonderful new superfood ingredients?"

1. Health Food and Organic Stores
2. Pharmacies / Drug Stores
3. Specialty Food Shops
4. Some Supermarkets – ask at your local supermarket
5. Websites – order from local businesses online
6. Amazon.com – or your country's Amazon website
7. Google – search for stores and products nearest to you

Until relatively recently, superfoods - in any form - have been enjoyed mainly by a small niche market of fans who stumbled across them, or had them recommended by a friend or family member. In the last few years, more supermarkets have begun putting their toe in the water by offering a small line of dried superfood products, which often seem to be located in an obscure corner of the supermarket.

Slowly but surely, superfoods are entering the mainstream consciousness; most people have heard the word 'superfoods' on television, or mentioned somewhere, but they haven't tried them and are probably still sceptical. Even if they *are* contemplating trying superfoods, they may not know where to start.

Supermarkets that *do* carry a selection of dried superfoods, may not carry every single one of the ones that we use in our recipes, and you'll probably need to ask an assistant where they are.

Most of the products we use should be available in your local Health Food or Organic Store. Stocking of certain ones may differ according to local regional differences and tastes. We recommend, using your phonebook to ring around and check first, before you trudge around town. Most health food businesses have a website, and checking this out first will save you time and shoe leather.

Donna sells her own personally blended superfood products 'exclusively online' to New Zealand and Australian customers, and there are probably similar online superfood stores in your country or region. Google is your friend; just try typing in the name of the product you're looking for and your location and hopefully you'll find what you're looking for nearby.

Since Donna's business is solely based down-under, the high cost of shipping generally makes it impractical and prohibitive to offer her products further afield than New Zealand and Australia.

If you live in the US, we recommend ordering via Amazon.com, if you don't have a preferred local supplier. Amazon makes it very easy. If you are based in the USA, it makes sense because ALL of the products we use are available on Amazon. You can order from the comfort of your own home, and their shipping costs are very reasonable within the US.

To help you choose from Amazon's huge range, Donna has selected a comparable matching superfood product on Amazon that she believes to be highest quality equivalent to her own range*. (See pg. 60 – 'Superfoods Descriptions + Info')

* NOTE: Because we don't *control* these products, we can't guarantee that all the Amazon links will continue to remain valid in the future.

If you don't want to shop online and you don't find a good local supplier on your first try, it may be a matter of persevering until you come across one you like.

We hope this advice helps you find a reliable source of superfoods locally. If not, reach out to us on Facebook and we'll try to help.

* * *

Conclusion

Try our 'Chocolate Pudding Challenge'...

Let's re-visit the question we posed earlier on pg.50 of this book, "Will 'superfoods' really help me be healthier and feel better?"

It is a good question. So, what's our answer?

It's tempting just to say, YES, they worked for me! But, for a more 'nutrient-dense' answer, let's look a little deeper at the quality of the food produced by our 'modern' food production methods.

Let's consider the vital relationship between our modern diet and our health. The steady and observable decline in health and rise of chronic conditions such as allergies, asthma, and skin conditions in western countries over the last 60-100 years is generally agreed by scientists and medical experts to be in large part attributable to changes in our diet.

What about other factors, like exercise?

The other biggest factor in this decline is undoubtedly the increasing trend of employment moving from outdoor, physical work to more sedentary occupations.

This takes us away from the best natural source of vitamin D (the sun) and regular exposure to rare, but necessary, elements such as selenium (from soil). This trend weakens our muscles (including the heart) and also weakens our immune system (from lack of exposure to bacterial challenges).

It also slows our metabolism, decreasing its efficiency to burn fats and other harmful elements in our food that would have, under our previously vigorous outdoor lifestyle, been burned up, utilised, or expelled by our bodies.

Can it all be attributed to our modern lifestyle?

The factors we touched on in the previous paragraph, combined with the fact that our lungs (with subsequent flow-on to our blood streams) are now more likely to be sucking in stale, unhealthy air (often) full of mould spores and germs into our bodies - rather than fresh air on a regular basis, show that our modern lifestyle is far less healthy than that of our grandparents or great-grandparents.

They probably worked outside and ate a lot of fresh, uncontaminated produce that they grew themselves, or at least had easy access to, in a way that most modern city-dwellers do not. What most modern city-dwellers *do* have easy access to, are lots of highly processed, packaged, nutrient-poor foods; full of added sugars, salts and fats; coloured and chemically enhanced to 'look' fresh. Yum, yum.

Ironically, advancements in medicine are keeping increasingly unhealthy, chronically sick people alive longer, to enjoy a poorer quality of life. That's our very broad overview of the modern diet and lifestyle in most 'western' countries; it seems to us to be becoming the reality for more and more people every day.

Thanks to the Internet, a growing awareness of these issues is spreading around the world and is leading to the strong realisation that we need to change our unhealthy eating lifestyles. We believe the rapid growth of the superfood community worldwide is also evidence of that. Unfortunately, *cost* shuts many out from healthier food and nutrition alternatives, including superfoods.

We've noticed the use of 'hype' in the marketing of certain 'trendy' superfoods…

Sadly, there are always some greedy or unscrupulous (or maybe even a few genuine, but ignorant) marketers who are willing to make extravagant claims around a particular ‘currently trendy’ superfood, in order to exploit the gullible, the vulnerable, and sometimes desperate people hoping for some miraculous cure for a serious health condition.

While superfoods can be helpful to many health conditions and will support the body in its fight to repair and heal itself, they’re best used long-term as part of a healthy lifestyle and balanced diet, for general health. They are unlikely to produce a miraculous effect on someone in the last stages of a major or life-threatening illness. Please consult your licensed medical practitioner for advice if you, or a loved one, are thinking of incorporating superfoods as part of a treatment program for any such condition.

However, for most people, there are many compelling reasons to consider adding superfoods to your diet. While sceptics remain, it is hard to deny the increasing wealth of anecdotal evidence for the benefits of incorporating superfoods into one’s diet.

On the simple principle of 'rubbish in, rubbish out' it logically makes sense that putting natural, raw, organic foods into our bodies will generally lead to a better functioning bodily system than consuming nutrient-poor, non-natural foods full of chemicals and additives, as well as added sugars and fats.

The Superfood trend reveals…

There is an emerging awareness among like-minded people who are choosing to eat better, think better and feel better by eating healthy, nutrient-rich foods. These are the people Donna has dubbed ‘superfoodies’; she coined this term to describe those who both love and are very knowledgeable about good food (foodies), but who also consider superfoods among the wisest and best ingredients to incorporate into the creation of good food.

* * *

Try our 'Chocolate Pudding' Challenge …

Isn't the proof always *in* the pudding?

So, why not give superfoods a try?

In our experience, most people find, after adding superfoods to their regular diet (often by simply replacing breakfast with a superfood smoothie), that they feel more energetic; they start noticing improvements in, or even the total elimination of, minor health irritations; that they're losing weight, or maintaining a healthy weight; and generally feeling more sustained and balanced.

Elsewhere in this book we've included some of the testimonials and stories (See pg.64) that Donna gets regularly from people using her 'Superfoodies' products. You can find tons of completely independent testimonials if you Google, 'testimonials about superfoods' (for example), to find loads more people reporting similar superfoods experiences all around the world.

You'll find all 21 recipes in this book delicious and easy-to-make, as well as being good for you and your loved ones.

We hope you enjoy them *all* and find yourself reaping the healthy rewards of superfoods, very soon.

Donna & Kay

PS. Don't forget you're not alone; there's a whole community of 'super foodies' travelling with you.

Please reach out to us via Facebook or email, if you need help making the recipes, or any other superfoods advice. We look forward to hearing about your journey.

FOLLOW :: Donna on Facebook :: Facebook.com/SuperFoodies

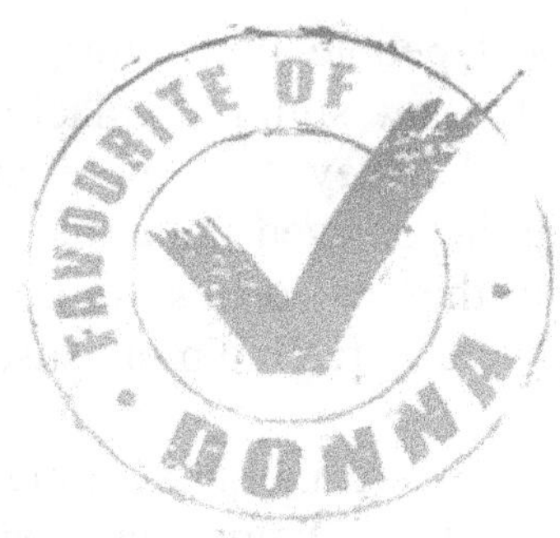

Still not sure which recipe to try first ?

We recommend you start with one of Donna's 'Top 3 Tick Start' recipes. They're the ones with this 'tick' icon.

They're on these pages :

1. **Hi-Antioxidant Berry Smoothie** >> TRY ME on pg.8
2. **Big Vit C Smoothie** >> TRY ME on pg.28
3. **Mango Smoothie** >> TRY ME on pg.26

Why not try one tonight?

But *before* you rush off to the kitchen …

▼

▼

▼

▼

▼

▼

The End

Except

▼

▼

▼

▼

▼

▼

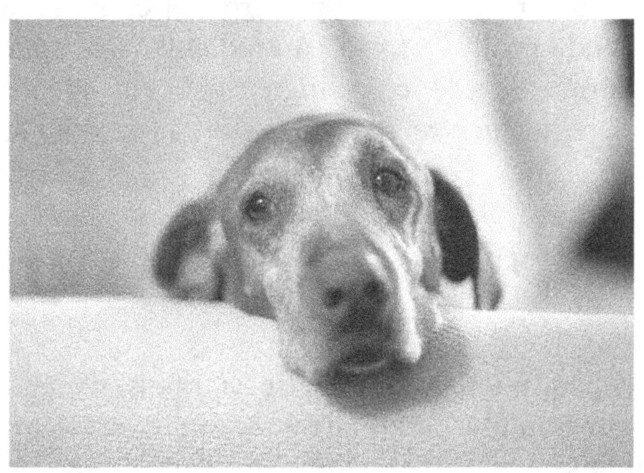

To thank *you* sincerely for buying our book!

<u>We really appreciate it.</u>

Would you be kind enough to help us make our next book *even* better ?

Please take a few minutes to give us your <u>honest</u> REVIEW on Amazon.com

Thanks so much!

Donna & Kay

Recipe Diary

Have superfood fun being 'experimental'...

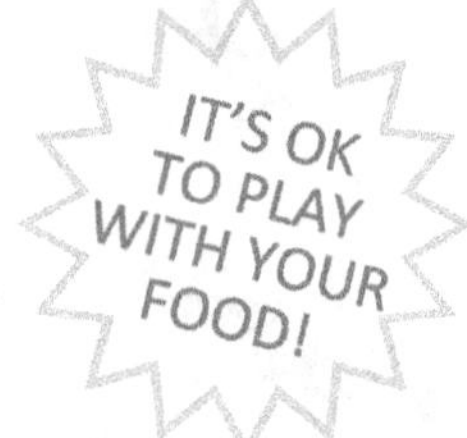

Why this Recipe Diary?

Donna's recipes are designed around a base of 'core' ingredients that she has carefully balanced to deliver *nutritional punch* and flavour. They are intentionally built from a combination of 'dried superfoods' and healthy fresh ingredients that allow you to experiment around these core ingredients, to create your own variations, adapting each recipe to your own personal tastes.

** Note: The '21 Best Superfood Smoothies' recipes are great to adapt because ideally you'll be using them a lot; it's good to have alternatives for variety and when there is seasonal un-availability of certain fresh ingredients.*

One day, Donna intends to release a book which specifically isolates the (absolutely essential) *core* ingredients in her recipes and highlighting which *optional* ingredients may be exchanged with others; without losing any of the targeted benefits and nutritional value.

But until that book comes out, why not conduct your own experiments to see what variations on Donna's recipes will work for you? Obviously, not *every* ingredient change will work, so you may have a misfire or two, but that's all part of the fun!

Donna does a lot of *experimenting* herself, and brings a lot of existing knowledge and years of experience to guide her, but balancing nutritional content with appropriate flavour combinations can be tricky sometimes. That's why 'tried and true' combinations are great starting points. Sometimes you may have to compromise on one thing in order to retain another. Some great flavour combinations are not necessarily as healthy or beneficial as others that may be less agreeable to the taste buds. The ideal result, of course, is to achieve the perfect balance of both.

Since Donna has done most of the work with these recipes, she recommends that you try your own experiments to find out if your own personal favourite will work - once you've given the originals a fair go, of course!

The best way to do this would be to change out only *one* of the fresh ingredients each time you make the recipe, and see what you think. Is it good? Does it taste terrible? Does it work with the other ingredients? Once you think you're on the right track, you could try adding one or two more new flavours with additional fresh ingredients. Don't forget to try some nuts or seeds, too.

Donna recommends you don't go 'overboard' with adding 'too many' new ingredients, because your body can only absorb so many good things in one go. You may be just wasting your money, time - and ingredients. That's why it's best to start with one change, then proceed up to two or three in total. If your experiments work, that will give you sufficient new options, without going crazy!

There will also be plenty of times when adaption, or experimentation, is absolutely necessary!

Sometimes this will be forced upon you by seasonal un-availability of fresh fruit and vegetables, or by the fact you simply forgot to replenish your pantry! It happens to the best of us. You've been busy rushing around all week and finally that birthday party or gathering of family or friends is suddenly upon you. You planned to delight everybody with your amazingly healthy chocolate treats, but when you rush to the pantry… shock, horror!… some key ingredient of a recipe is missing! Maybe more than one. You've got literally, 'no time' to replenish them, so you're forced to adapt and try to find something new to replace what is missing.

That's a great reason, for trying a few 'experiments', with ingredient variations, long *before* you find yourself in that dire situation.

It's not such a daunting prospect if you already *know* that certain flavour combinations are successful, and you already understand how to 'balance' different flavour 'profiles' against each other. 'Tried and true' is only that way because, back down the track, someone tried experimenting until they got it right! You don't want find yourself experimenting on your guests, and hoping it's not a disaster!

So, after you've given the existing recipes a good and thorough try-out (which should keep you busy for a while), use these Diary pages to keep track of your 'experiments'. Record the details here.

Don't just rely on your memory, especially in a moment of panic. It's much better to come back to your notes, in your very own handwriting, in this section of the book, and confirm what your memory is telling you.

How to use this Recipe Diary:

1. Have Fun by Experimenting with Donna's Recipes.
2. Record the results in this Recipe Diary.
3. Change-out one of the recipe ingredients (fresh is easiest).
4. If you like the new change, either stop there or continue.
5. Add/change, up to 2 more additional ingredients.
6. Record your changes, and thoughts on the results in 'Notes'.
7. Rate your Experiment out of 7, and then circle either:
   Yes – No – Maybe.

Go and have lots of fun. Happy experimenting!

Experiment #1

Recipe Notes:

Don't rely on your memory! Fill in *all* the details here and you'll always know exactly what you did - and if it worked or not.

Date: ....

Recipe Name: ....

Change #1:

Change #2:

Change #3:

*My Results:

Rate the Result: [Circle the number you believe to be the fairest.]

| 1 | 2 | 3 | 4 | 5 | 6 | 7 |

* Don't forget to record what you learn about different flavour combos. Could the new flavour work in a different recipe, or combination? Could it work with the addition of a balancing flavour/or flavours? If any other *inspired* ideas occur as you go, note them down for future experiments.

Circle one: YES! NO! MAYBE?

Experiment #2

Recipe Notes:

Don't rely on your memory! Fill in *all* the details here and you'll always know exactly what you did - and if it worked or not.

Date: ....

Recipe Name: ....

Change #1:

Change #2:

Change #3:

*My Results:

Rate the Result: [Circle the number you believe to be the fairest.]

1	2	3	4	5	6	7

* Don't forget to record what you learn about different flavour combos. Could the new flavour work in a different recipe, or combination? Could it work with the addition of a balancing flavour/or flavours? If any other *inspired* ideas occur as you go, note them down for future experiments.

Circle one: YES! NO! MAYBE?

Experiment #3

Recipe Notes:

Don't rely on your memory! Fill in *all* the details here and you'll always know exactly what you did - and if it worked or not.

Date: ....

Recipe Name: ....

Change #1: ______________________________

Change #2: ______________________________

Change #3: ______________________________

*My Results: ______________________________

____

____

____

Rate the Result: [Circle the number you believe to be the fairest.]

| 1 | 2 | 3 | 4 | 5 | 6 | 7 |

* Don't forget to record what you learn about different flavour combos. Could the new flavour work in a different recipe, or combination? Could it work with the addition of a balancing flavour/or flavours? If any other *inspired* ideas occur as you go, note them down for future experiments.

Circle one: YES! NO! MAYBE?

Experiment #4

Recipe Notes:

Don't rely on your memory! Fill in *all* the details here and you'll always know exactly what you did - and if it worked or not.

Date: ....

Recipe Name: ....

Change #1: ____________________

Change #2: ____________________

Change #3: ____________________

*My Results: ____________________

Rate the Result: [Circle the number you believe to be the fairest.]

| 1 | 2 | 3 | 4 | 5 | 6 | 7 |

* Don't forget to record what you learn about different flavour combos. Could the new flavour work in a different recipe, or combination? Could it work with the addition of a balancing flavour/or flavours? If any other *inspired* ideas occur as you go, note them down for future experiments.

Circle one: YES! NO! MAYBE?

Experiment #5

Recipe Notes:

Don't rely on your memory! Fill in *all* the details here and you'll always know exactly what you did - and if it worked or not.

Date: ....

Recipe Name: ....

Change #1: ____________________

Change #2: ____________________

Change #3: ____________________

*My Results: ____________________

Rate the Result: [Circle the number you believe to be the fairest.]

| 1 | 2 | 3 | 4 | 5 | 6 | 7 |

* Don't forget to record what you learn about different flavour combos. Could the new flavour work in a different recipe, or combination? Could it work with the addition of a balancing flavour/or flavours? If any other *inspired* ideas occur as you go, note them down for future experiments.

Circle one: YES! NO! MAYBE?

Experiment #6

Recipe Notes:

Don't rely on your memory! Fill in *all* the details here and you'll always know exactly what you did - and if it worked or not.

Date: ....

Recipe Name: ....

Change #1:

Change #2:

Change #3:

*My Results:

Rate the Result: [Circle the number you believe to be the fairest.]

| 1 | 2 | 3 | 4 | 5 | 6 | 7 |

* Don't forget to record what you learn about different flavour combos. Could the new flavour work in a different recipe, or combination? Could it work with the addition of a balancing flavour/or flavours? If any other *inspired* ideas occur as you go, note them down for future experiments.

Circle one: YES! NO! MAYBE?

Experiment #7

Recipe Notes:

Don't rely on your memory! Fill in *all* the details here and you'll always know exactly what you did - and if it worked or not.

Date: ....

Recipe Name: ....

Change #1:

Change #2:

Change #3:

*My Results:

Rate the Result: [Circle the number you believe to be the fairest.]

| 1 | 2 | 3 | 4 | 5 | 6 | 7 |

* Don't forget to record what you learn about different flavour combos. Could the new flavour work in a different recipe, or combination? Could it work with the addition of a balancing flavour/or flavours? If any other *inspired* ideas occur as you go, note them down for future experiments.

Circle one: YES! NO! MAYBE?

Experiment #8

Recipe Notes:

Don't rely on your memory! Fill in *all* the details here and you'll always know exactly what you did - and if it worked or not.

Date: ………………………………

Recipe Name: ……………………………………………………..……

Change #1: ____

Change #2: ____

Change #3: ____

*My Results: ____

Rate the Result: [Circle the number you believe to be the fairest.]

| 1 | 2 | 3 | 4 | 5 | 6 | 7 |

* Don't forget to record what you learn about different flavour combos. Could the new flavour work in a different recipe, or combination? Could it work with the addition of a balancing flavour/or flavours? If any other *inspired* ideas occur as you go, note them down for future experiments.

Circle one: YES! NO! MAYBE?

Experiment #9

Recipe Notes:

Don't rely on your memory! Fill in *all* the details here and you'll always know exactly what you did - and if it worked or not.

Date: ....

Recipe Name: ....……

Change #1: ______________________

Change #2: ______________________

Change #3: ______________________

*My Results: ______________________

____

____

____

Rate the Result: [Circle the number you believe to be the fairest.]

| 1 | 2 | 3 | 4 | 5 | 6 | 7 |

* Don't forget to record what you learn about different flavour combos. Could the new flavour work in a different recipe, or combination? Could it work with the addition of a balancing flavour/or flavours? If any other *inspired* ideas occur as you go, note them down for future experiments.

Circle one: YES! NO! MAYBE?

Experiment #10

Recipe Notes:

Don't rely on your memory! Fill in *all* the details here and you'll always know exactly what you did - and if it worked or not.

Date: ....

Recipe Name: ....

Change #1: ____________________________

Change #2: ____________________________

Change #3: ____________________________

*My Results: ____________________________

Rate the Result: [Circle the number you believe to be the fairest.]

| 1 | 2 | 3 | 4 | 5 | 6 | 7 |

* <u>Don't</u> forget to record what you learn about different flavour combos. Could the new flavour work in a different recipe, or combination? Could it work with the addition of a balancing flavour/or flavours? If any other *inspired* ideas occur as you go, note them down for future experiments.

Circle one: YES! NO! MAYBE?

Experiment #11

Recipe Notes:

Don't rely on your memory! Fill in *all* the details here and you'll always know exactly what you did - and if it worked or not.

Date: ....

Recipe Name: ....

Change #1: ______________________

Change #2: ______________________

Change #3: ______________________

*My Results: ______________________

Rate the Result: [Circle the number you believe to be the fairest.]

| 1 | 2 | 3 | 4 | 5 | 6 | 7 |

* Don't forget to record what you learn about different flavour combos. Could the new flavour work in a different recipe, or combination? Could it work with the addition of a balancing flavour/or flavours? If any other *inspired* ideas occur as you go, note them down for future experiments.

Circle one: YES! NO! MAYBE?

Experiment #12

Recipe Notes:

Don't rely on your memory! Fill in *all* the details here and you'll always know exactly what you did - and if it worked or not.

Date: ....

Recipe Name: ....

Change #1:

Change #2:

Change #3:

*My Results:

Rate the Result: [Circle the number you believe to be the fairest.]

| 1 | 2 | 3 | 4 | 5 | 6 | 7 |

* Don't forget to record what you learn about different flavour combos. Could the new flavour work in a different recipe, or combination? Could it work with the addition of a balancing flavour/or flavours? If any other *inspired* ideas occur as you go, note them down for future experiments.

Circle one: YES! NO! MAYBE?

Experiment #13

Recipe Notes:

Don't rely on your memory! Fill in *all* the details here and you'll always know exactly what you did - and if it worked or not.

Date: ....

Recipe Name: ....

Change #1: ______________________________

Change #2: ______________________________

Change #3: ______________________________

*My Results: ______________________________

____

____

____

Rate the Result: [Circle the number you believe to be the fairest.]

| 1 | 2 | 3 | 4 | 5 | 6 | 7 |

* Don't forget to record what you learn about different flavour combos. Could the new flavour work in a different recipe, or combination? Could it work with the addition of a balancing flavour/or flavours? If any other *inspired* ideas occur as you go, note them down for future experiments.

Circle one: YES! NO! MAYBE?

Experiment #14

Recipe Notes:

Don't rely on your memory! Fill in *all* the details here and you'll always know exactly what you did - and if it worked or not.

Date: ....

Recipe Name: ....

Change #1:

Change #2:

Change #3:

*My Results:

Rate the Result: [Circle the number you believe to be the fairest.]

| 1 | 2 | 3 | 4 | 5 | 6 | 7 |

* <u>Don't</u> forget to record what you learn about different flavour combos. Could the new flavour work in a different recipe, or combination? Could it work with the addition of a balancing flavour/or flavours? If any other *inspired* ideas occur as you go, note them down for future experiments.

Circle one: YES! NO! MAYBE?

Experiment #15

Recipe Notes:

Don't rely on your memory! Fill in *all* the details here and you'll always know exactly what you did - and if it worked or not.

Date: ………………………………

Recipe Name: ……………………………………………………..……

Change #1:

Change #2:

Change #3:

*My Results:

Rate the Result: [Circle the number you believe to be the fairest.]

| 1 | 2 | 3 | 4 | 5 | 6 | 7 |

* Don't forget to record what you learn about different flavour combos. Could the new flavour work in a different recipe, or combination? Could it work with the addition of a balancing flavour/or flavours? If any other *inspired* ideas occur as you go, note them down for future experiments.

Circle one: YES! NO! MAYBE?

Experiment #16

Recipe Notes:

Don't rely on your memory! Fill in *all* the details here and you'll always know exactly what you did - and if it worked or not.

Date: ....

Recipe Name: ....

Change #1:

Change #2:

Change #3:

*My Results:

Rate the Result: [Circle the number you believe to be the fairest.]

| 1 | 2 | 3 | 4 | 5 | 6 | 7 |

* Don't forget to record what you learn about different flavour combos. Could the new flavour work in a different recipe, or combination? Could it work with the addition of a balancing flavour/or flavours? If any other *inspired* ideas occur as you go, note them down for future experiments.

Circle one: YES! NO! MAYBE?

Experiment #17

Recipe Notes:

Don't rely on your memory! Fill in *all* the details here and you'll always know exactly what you did - and if it worked or not.

Date: ………………………………

Recipe Name: ……………………………………………………

Change #1:

Change #2:

Change #3:

*My Results:

Rate the Result: [Circle the number you believe to be the fairest.]

| 1 | 2 | 3 | 4 | 5 | 6 | 7 |

* Don't forget to record what you learn about different flavour combos. Could the new flavour work in a different recipe, or combination? Could it work with the addition of a balancing flavour/or flavours? If any other *inspired* ideas occur as you go, note them down for future experiments.

Circle one: YES! NO! MAYBE?

Experiment #18

Recipe Notes:

Don't rely on your memory! Fill in *all* the details here and you'll always know exactly what you did - and if it worked or not.

Date: ....

Recipe Name: ....

Change #1:

Change #2:

Change #3:

*My Results:

Rate the Result: [Circle the number you believe to be the fairest.]

| 1 | 2 | 3 | 4 | 5 | 6 | 7 |

* Don't forget to record what you learn about different flavour combos. Could the new flavour work in a different recipe, or combination? Could it work with the addition of a balancing flavour/or flavours? If any other *inspired* ideas occur as you go, note them down for future experiments.

Circle one: YES! NO! MAYBE?

Experiment #19

Recipe Notes:

Don't rely on your memory! Fill in *all* the details here and you'll always know exactly what you did - and if it worked or not.

Date: ....

Recipe Name: ....

Change #1:

Change #2:

Change #3:

*My Results:

Rate the Result: [Circle the number you believe to be the fairest.]

| 1 | 2 | 3 | 4 | 5 | 6 | 7 |

* Don't forget to record what you learn about different flavour combos. Could the new flavour work in a different recipe, or combination? Could it work with the addition of a balancing flavour/or flavours? If any other *inspired* ideas occur as you go, note them down for future experiments.

Circle one: YES! NO! MAYBE?

Experiment #20

Recipe Notes:

Don't rely on your memory! Fill in *all* the details here and you'll always know exactly what you did - and if it worked or not.

Date: ………………………………

Recipe Name: …………………………………………………...……

Change #1:

Change #2:

Change #3:

*My Results:

Rate the Result: [Circle the number you believe to be the fairest.]

| 1 | 2 | 3 | 4 | 5 | 6 | 7 |

* <u>Don't</u> forget to record what you learn about different flavour combos. Could the new flavour work in a different recipe, or combination? Could it work with the addition of a balancing flavour/or flavours? If any other *inspired* ideas occur as you go, note them down for future experiments.

Circle one: YES! NO! MAYBE?

Experiment #21

Recipe Notes:

Don't rely on your memory! Fill in *all* the details here and you'll always know exactly what you did - and if it worked or not.

Date: ....

Recipe Name: ....

Change #1: ____________________

Change #2: ____________________

Change #3: ____________________

*My Results: ____________________

____

____

____

Rate the Result: [Circle the number you believe to be the fairest.]

| 1 | 2 | 3 | 4 | 5 | 6 | 7 |

* Don't forget to record what you learn about different flavour combos. Could the new flavour work in a different recipe, or combination? Could it work with the addition of a balancing flavour/or flavours? If any other *inspired* ideas occur as you go, note them down for future experiments.

Circle one: YES! NO! MAYBE?

Don't forget...

1. Your 3 Free Bonus Berry Brain-food Recipes!

Type this into your Internet browser >
www.superfoodies.co.nz/book2free

2. Our other Amazon books.

Book #1: '21 Best Superfood Cacao Recipes'
Go here >> www.amazon.com/dp/B0178USZ88

Book #3: '21 Best Brain-food Berry Recipes'
Go here >> www.amazon.com/dp/B01LWJLKOD

3. Please help us – with an honest review ...

We write our books with *you* in mind. Please take 5 minutes to give us your honest REVIEW on Amazon. Tell us what you like about our book(s) – and where we can improve for you, in future editions.

Review here >> www.amazon.com/dp/B01J73OAKG

Still turning pages?

Why?

Are you expecting a big …

Surprise!

EXTRA BONUS RECIPE from our New Book #3

Book #3 – '21 Best Berry Brain-food Recipes'
Out now on Amazon.com

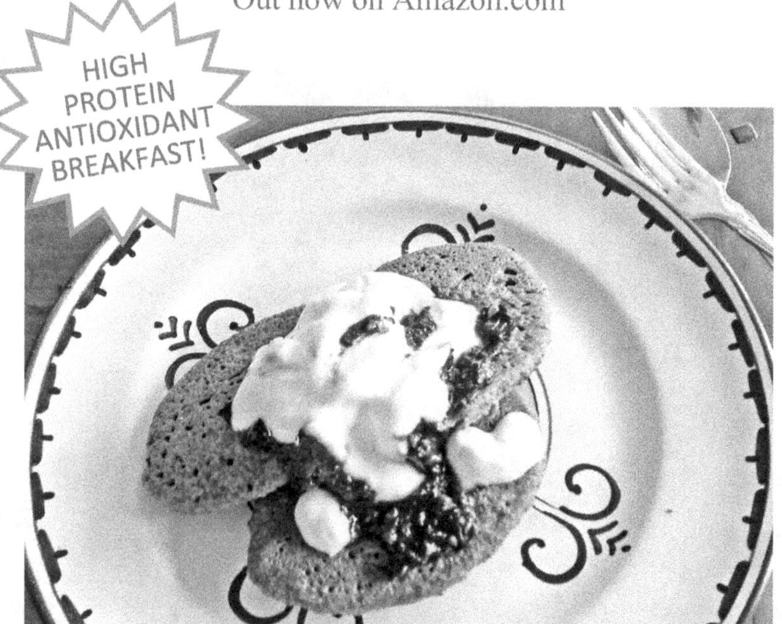

Acai Berry Hotcakes

Serving size: makes 9 hotcakes
Time to make: 30 minutes

Ingredients for Hot Cakes

2 teaspoons acai berry powder
1 tablespoon lucuma powder
¼ cup chia seeds
1 cup whole buckwheat
1-2 teaspoons baking powder
1 pinch of salt
1¾ cups filtered water

Ingredients for Berry Sauce

1 cup frozen / or fresh boysenberries
3 prunes
1-2 teaspoons acai berry powder

Hot Cakes Method

1. Place all ingredients except water in blender and start processing on low speed.
2. Gradually add water while processing and then blitz to a smooth creamy batter.
3. Heat a non-stick frying pan. Use a little coconut oil to wipe pan if preferred.
4. Ladle batter into frying pan in heaped tablespoon measurements.
5. Cook hotcakes a couple of minutes until small holes appear, then turn them over in pan to cook other side. These hotcakes are easy to turn over.
6. Put aside and keep warm until ready to eat.

Berry Sauce Method

1. Place berries and prunes in saucepan on top of stove.
2. Heat on low heat until prunes are very soft and berries collapsed.
3. Remove from heat and mix until prunes are blended and berries are broken up.
4. Finally mix in acai berry powder and beat to preferred consistency.
5. Serve hotcakes with this antioxidant charged berry sauce and some coconut yoghurt.

* Notes:

Start the berry sauce first, so that the berries are slowly condensing while you make the hotcakes. This is a high protein, antioxidant charged breakfast.

* * *

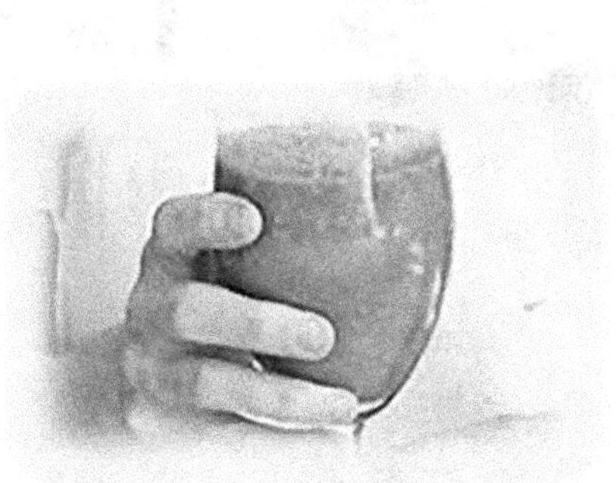

"Drinking smoothies is a fun, delicious way to boost your health."

– Donna.

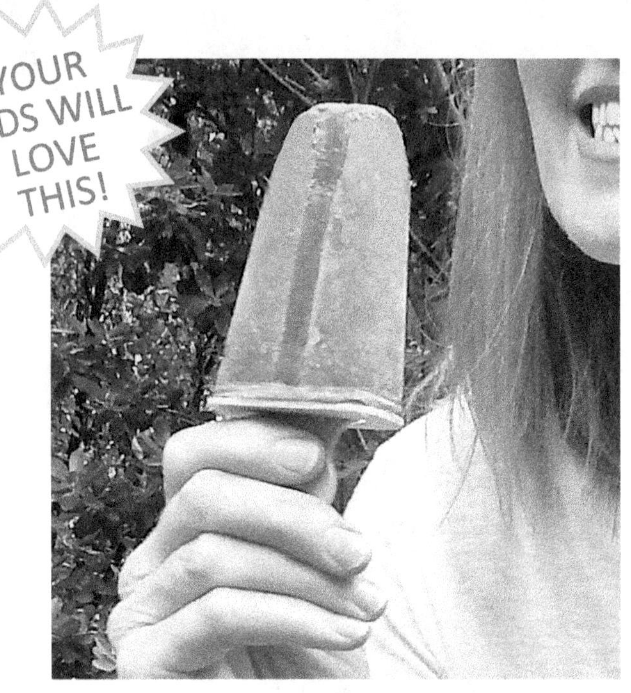

Surprise your kids this summer…

Turn my superfood smoothies into delicious, healthy popsicles.

Your kids will love them! They're yummy, flavour-packed 'superfood popsicles' - ideal for hot summer days.

Or *anytime* you feel like a cool treat.

They're ridiculously *easy* to make …

Just pour your liquid smoothies into popsicle molds and 'pop' them in your freezer overnight, or until solid. Simple as 1,2,3 …

1. Make your favourite smoothie.
2. Pour into a popsicle mold.
3. Place in freezer until solid.

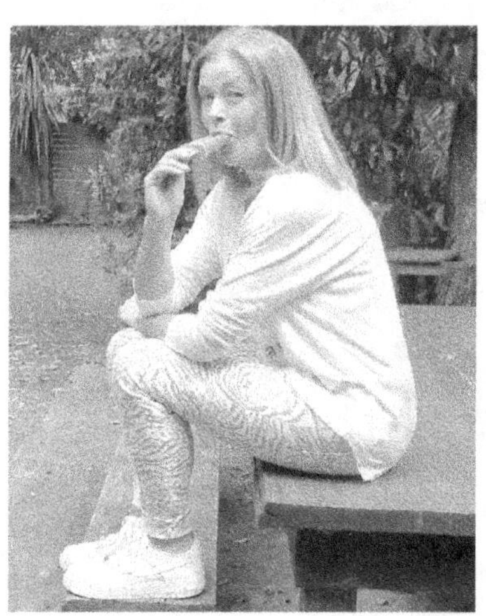

Then, treat your family and friends to the healthiest, tastiest popsicle they've probably ever eaten!

Kids love berry and fruit smoothie popsicles best - because they're flavour-packed and super delicious. And they won't even know they are healthy! These popsicles are a great way to avoid the sugary, unhealthy ice-creams and cordial-based alternatives.

Where can you find popsicle molds?

Popsicle molds are cheap – from $10 to $20 US – and can be purchased from a zillion retailers from Walmart to Kmart.

You can order them online from Amazon, too.

For example, below is just one we found on Amazon with a quick search for 'popsicle molds'.

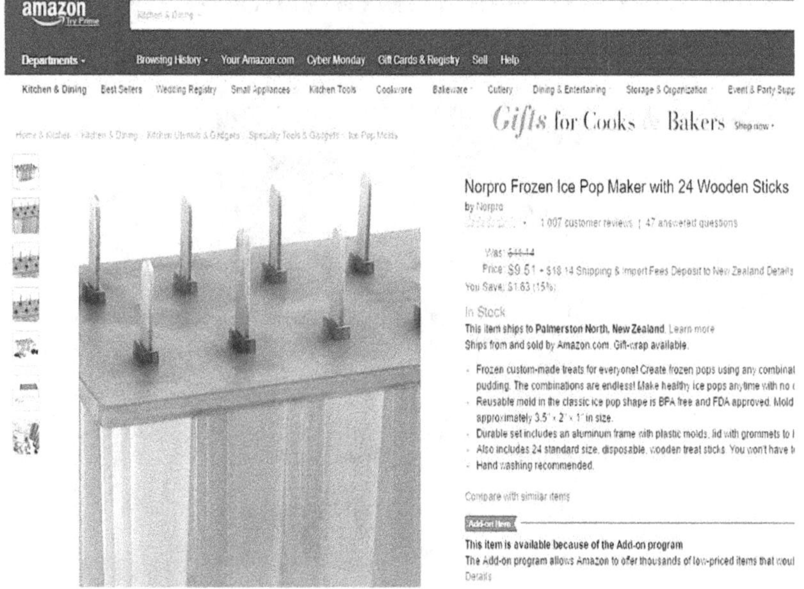

Here's the Amazon link to the above:
www.amazon.com/gp/product/B0002IBJOG

However, once you go there you will see links to a wide array of other choices below that product. Or, just do your own search for 'popsicle molds' in Amazon's search box.

Here are just a *few* different kinds of popsicle molds available …

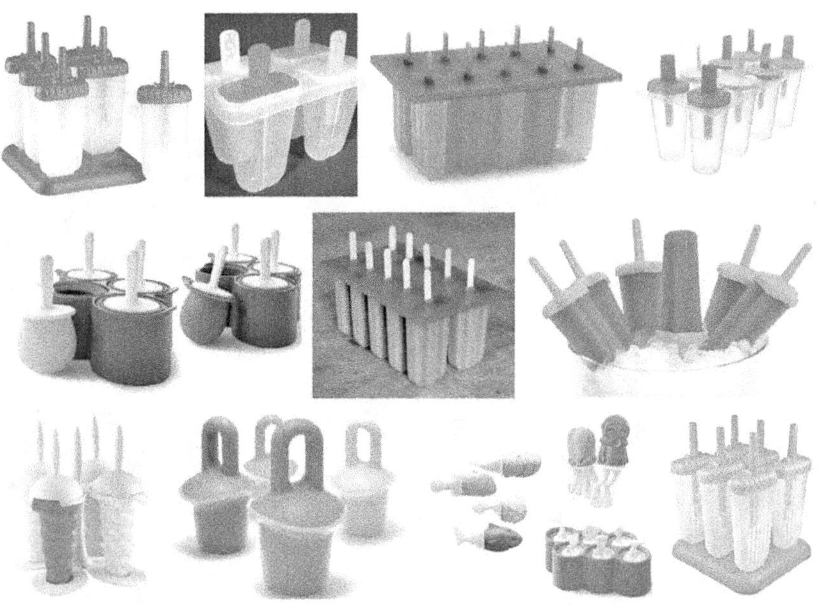

The screenshot above shows a small selection of the different popsicle molds on the market. These are from Amazom.com but you can find a huge variety at other retailers, like Walmart.

Popsicle molds come in lots of colourful shapes and sizes that your kids will love. Plus, they'll make your 'healthy popsicles' even *more* fun to eat!

Be aware:

Some molds come with sticks attached (silicone/plastic) and some use wooden sticks you'll need to buy more of when the supplied ones run out.

* * *

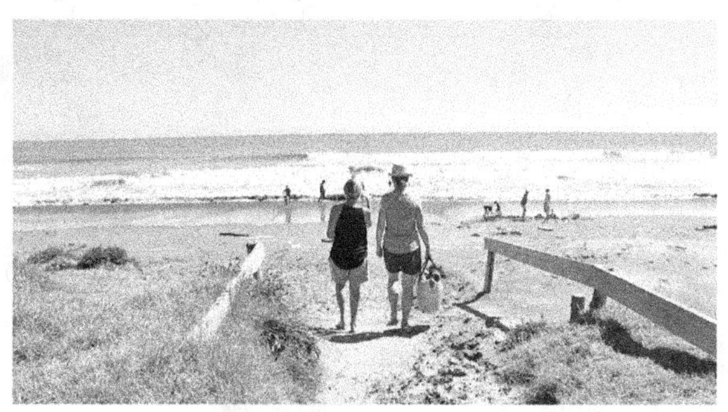

Bye, for now,

We're off to the beach.
See you in our next book.

-Donna & Kay.

:: End ::

Books by Donna & Kay

The Discover Superfoods Series – *by* Donna Davidson and Kay Wood.

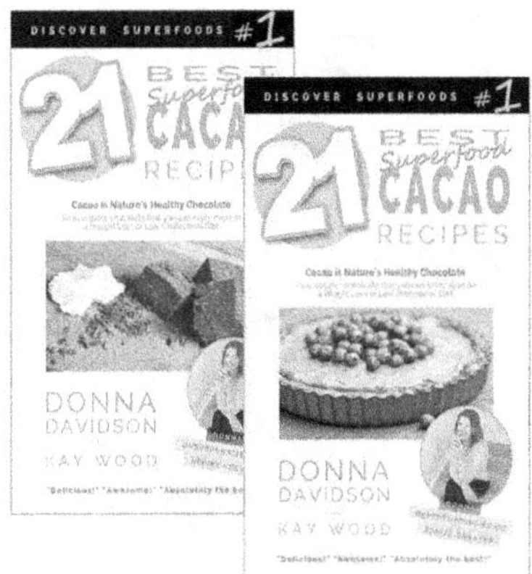

KINDLE / eBook
Discover Superfoods Book #1
21 Best Superfood Cacao Recipes
Available on Amazon.

PRINT BOOK
Discover Superfoods Book #1
21 Best Superfood Cacao Recipes
Available on Amazon.

* * * * * * * * * * * * * * *

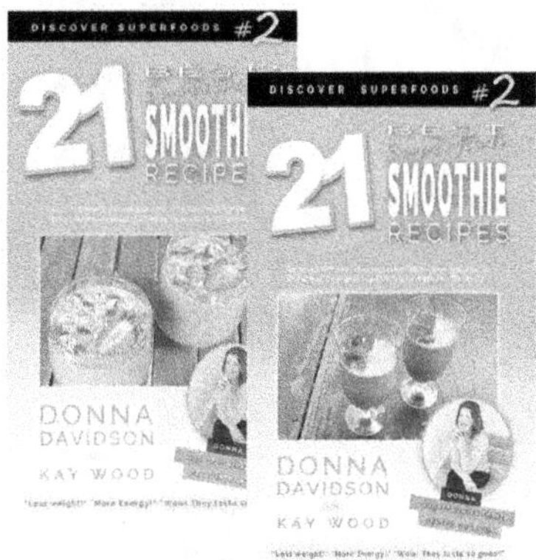

KINDLE / eBook
Discover Superfoods Book #2
21 Best Superfood Smoothie Recipes
Available on Amazon

PRINT BOOK
Discover Superfoods Book #2
21 Best Superfood Smoothie Recipes
Available on Amazon

* * * * * * * * * * * * * * *

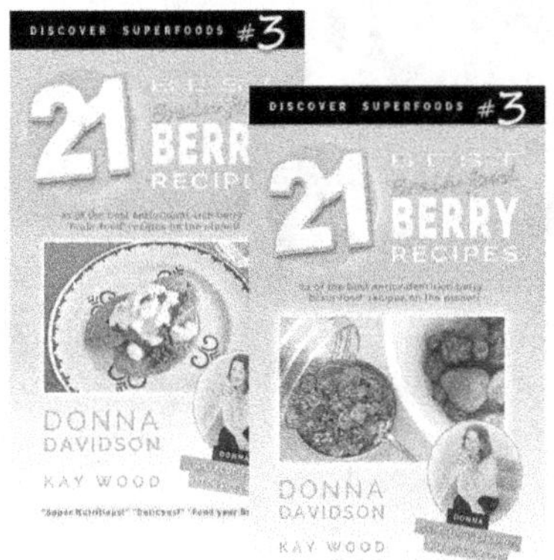

KINDLE / eBook
Discover Superfoods Book #3
21 Best Berry Brain-food Recipes
Available on Amazon

PRINT BOOK
Discover Superfoods Book #3
21 Best Berry Brain-food Recipes
Available on Amazon

The Secret to better health?

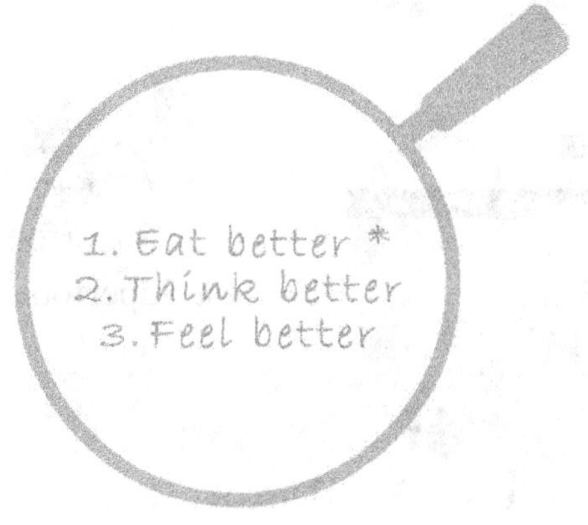

"Good food is better medicine than medicine. If you enjoy the privilege of being able to choose to eat better, you are among the lucky ones. Make that choice today and save on your future medical bills, mental anguish, physical pain, and years of living with a lower quality of life than you needed to."

- D&K.

www.ingramcontent.com/pod-product-compliance
Lightning Source LLC
Chambersburg PA
CBHW050349280326
41933CB00010BA/1390

9780473367305